The International Library

THE NATURE OF
INTELLIGENCE

Founded by C. K. Ogden

The International Library of Psychology

INDIVIDUAL DIFFERENCES
In 21 Volumes

THE NATURE OF
INTELLIGENCE

L L THURSTONE

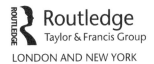

Routledge
Taylor & Francis Group
LONDON AND NEW YORK

First published in 1924 by
Routledge, Trench, Trubner & Co., Ltd.
2 Park Square, Milton Park, Abingdon, Oxfordshire OX14 4RN
711 Third Avenue, New York, NY 10017

First issued in paperback 2014

Routledge is an imprint of the Taylor and Francis Group, an informa business

The publishers have made every effort to contact authors/copyright holders
of the works reprinted in the *International Library of Psychology*.
This has not been possible in every case, however, and we would
welcome correspondence from those individuals/companies
we have been unable to trace.

These reprints are taken from original copies of each book. In many cases
the condition of these originals is not perfect. The publisher has gone to
great lengths to ensure the quality of these reprints, but wishes to point
out that certain characteristics of the original copies will, of necessity, be
apparent in reprints thereof.

British Library Cataloguing in Publication Data
A CIP catalogue record for this book
is available from the British Library

The Nature of Intelligence
ISBN 0415-21069-0
Individual Differences: 21 Volumes
ISBN 0415-21130-1
The International Library of Psychology: 204 Volumes
ISBN 0415-19132-7

ISBN 13: 978-1-138-88255-3 (pbk)
ISBN 13: 978-0-415-21069-0 (hbk)

TO

MY FATHER AND MOTHER

CONTENTS

PREFACE

SINCE the book-market has been flooded with psycho-analysis, it is of some interest to inquire into the relation between the points of view that psychoanalysis represents and the points of view that the older schools of psychology have adopted in the interpretation of mind. Psychoanalytic theory is strange and extreme, to be sure, both in the technical journals devoted to its professional discussion and in the popular books on the subject. But there is an underlying truth in the psychoanalytic literature which can be extracted from the strange context, and which has not been adequately noted in the more established scientific studies of mind.

The contrast between abnormal psychology and normal psychology is, in this particular regard, very striking. The study of abnormal psychology radiates largely from the central question of discovering what satisfactions the patient is trying to attain, and how it comes about that he attempts to gain these satisfactions in the particular ways that we, as outsiders, consider to be ineffective and erratic. Our interest is in the patient, and we try to see his environment as it really looks to him. We discover, usually, that the satisfactions that the patient is trying to attain are universal for all of us, but we discover also that he is less successful than we are in using that environment.

When we turn to normal psychology we have an entirely different state of affairs. No longer are we mainly interested in what the normal person is trying to do, and the satisfactions that he is trying to attain. On the contrary, we describe the normal person in scientific psychology as though he were nothing more than a responding machine. In fact, the person who lends himself and his mind to the purposes of any experiment in a psychological laboratory is technically known as " the reagent ", and everything that he does and says is technically known as his " responses " or " reactions ". There is no fault to be found with this point of view for certain types of experimental work, but serious fault is to be found with the assumption that this point of view is at all adequate for psychology as a science.

In abnormal psychology we have, as I have said, the main emphasis placed on the patient and the exploration of his innermost self. His environment is looked upon merely as the means that happen to be available for him to satisfy his wants. We describe his erratic behaviour as the by-paths, substitutions, anomalies, and distortions that come about because of his repeated failure. We find that the patient is occasionally able so to distort his attitudes that he finds a compensatory kind of satisfaction in what seems to us queer conduct. He does attain satisfactions, however, even though he must distort his own attitudes toward life, his own sense organs and mental powers. Note that the cause-and-effect relations of such a psychological point of view start with the person himself, and that they terminate in the behaviour that satisfies him. This point of view reaches its most emphatic expression in psychoanalysis, and the fundamental truth about it that has been neglected in scientific psychology is that *action originates in the actor himself.*

When Jung's word-association test is given to a patient, the interest of the examiner is focussed on the patient in an attempt to learn what constitutes *his* desires, *his* failures, and *his* compromises with failure. But when we turn to the field of normal psychology, we find that in closely analogous experimentation the examiner is primarily interested in the *stimulus* and in the so-called *responses,* instead of in the *person.* The corresponding problems in normal psychology deal with the attempt to discover what fractional part of a second is required to perceive a word or to make a response, what particular arrangements in the stimulus facilitate or inhibit recall, and the effect that all sorts of variations in the stimulus can have on the response. The experimenter is then interested in describing the behaviour as in the nature of a response, and he attempts to describe the stimulus as the primary cause of the response. Normal psychology assumes that *action begins in the environment,* whereas abnormal psychology more often implies that *action begins in the actor himself.*

The point of view that is implied in abnormal psychology, according to which conduct has its root and starting-point in ourselves, is in better harmony with the other sciences that concern human nature. It is certainly easier for the preacher, the judge, and the teacher, to accept a system of psychology according to which conduct springs from man's inner self than to assimilate a psychological interpretation according to which we become reduced to reflex response machines that continually react to a fortuitous environment. The study of ethics, criminology, and sociology is certainly made more illuminating by a psychology that looks to the inner self as the mainspring of conduct and according to which the stimuli of the environment become merely the avenues through which that inner self is expressed and satisfied. It is just this point of view in the interpretation of human nature that psychoanalysis has emphasized, and that is primarily the reason why it has found popularity as an explanatory method in that large field of phenomena which is dominated by human nature. It is this shift of interest from the *stimulus-response relation to the wants of the living self* that marks the fundamental difference between what we know as the old and the new psychology.

It is by no means necessary to assume that the starting-point of action be a soul. It might as well be the energy released by the metabolism of the organism. It is pretty certain that with the advance of scientific psychology we shall come close to this kind of source for human conduct, and it may then turn out to be merely a more materialistic and dynamic equivalent of what has been vaguely called the soul or the self. It is certainly a fact that the so-called New Psychology falls readily into line with the other sciences of human nature in a way which has never been attained by the more established stimulus-response point of view.

Another psychological subject that is at the present time very much in the public mind is that of Intelligence Tests. Most of the psychological tests that are in common use have been arrived at principally by trying different tests for different purposes until certain tests have been found to be successful. There is considerable difference of opinion as to what intelligence really is, but, even if we do not know just what intelligence is, we can still use the tests as long as they are demonstrably satisfactory for definite practical ends. We use electricity for practical purposes even though we have been uncertain as to its ultimate nature, and it is so with the intelligence tests. We use the tests and leave it for separate inquiry to determine the ultimate nature of intelligence.

In these chapters I have started with the assumption that conduct originates in the actor himself, and I have tried to discover what intelligent conduct may mean if we follow this assumption to its limits. I find that the disparity between the new psychology, and the academic or scientific psychology and the most rigorously objective behaviourism breaks down completely. These three schools of psychological interpretation form a continuum, in that conduct originates in the self as studied by *psychiatry*, it takes partial and tentative formulations in conscious states as studied by *academic psychology*, and it completes itself into behaviour, as studied by the *behaviourist* school. The cognitive categories of academic psychology become, in such an interpretation, the incomplete and tentative formulations of conduct. Consciousness is interpreted as conduct which is in the process of being formed.

Intelligence is defined, according to this point of view, as the capacity to live a trial-and-error existence with alternatives that are as yet only incomplete conduct. To think is to cut and try with alternatives that are not yet fully formed into behaviour. The degree of intelligence is measured by the incompleteness of the alternatives which participate in the trial-and-error life of the actor. A concept becomes, then, an incomplete act, a small piece or derivative of conduct which anticipates the whole conduct. By its reference to the expected completion of the act it participates effectively in the trial-and-error expression of our wants. It is in this sense that intelligence and the capacity for abstraction are identical.

Psychology deals with a circuit which may be divided into four phases. It starts with the *life-impulses* in the organism. The next phase is the partial expression of these impulses which we know as *consciousness*. In that phase the life-impulses constitute the indices of expected experience in which the details of the expected conduct have not yet been filled in. The third phase consists in the *overt conduct* by which the life-impulses are registered on the environment. The fourth phase brings us back again into the organism in the form of *satisfactions*. The satisfactions are partly physical and partly social. Intelligence concerns the control that the organism exercises over the effectiveness and the balance of future satisfactions.

It may be that these chapters contain nothing that is fundamentally new beyond the attempt to harmonize three schools of thought about human nature which have the appearance of being irreconcilably disparate. Stated in a nutshell, my message is that *psychology starts with the unrest of the inner self, and it completes its discovery in the contentment of the inner self.*

I may conclude by expressing my indebtedness to my teachers, colleagues, and students for their influence on my psychological thought. To President Angell I am grateful for the introduction to the study of psychology which, by his influence, I chose as my life work. I believe that it was in Professor G. H. Mead's lectures on Social Psychology that I first started the line of thought from which the present book has developed, but I am quite sure that he would never recognize his own lectures as the source. The unusual scientific leadership of Professor W. V. Bingham is responsible for my efforts to reconcile the demands of practical psychology and of systematic method. I desire further to acknowledge the many ideas which I have derived from discussion with my colleagues, Professor David R. Craig, Dr. Max Schoen, Miss Thelma Gwinn, and Miss Esther Gatewood. My graduate students have removed numerous ambiguities by their criticism. The appreciative mention of all these people does not of course imply that they endorse my contentions.

L. L. THURSTONE.

PITTSBURG, PA.
    January, 1923.

CHAPTER I

THE STIMULUS-RESPONSE FALLACY IN PSYCHOLOGY[1]

1. THE OLD AND THE NEW PSYCHOLOGY

There has lately come into prominence before the reading public what is known as the New Psychology. This so-called new psychology is concerned with a wide variety of mental phenomena which have a strong interest appeal to every intelligent person. It purports to explain to us our dreams, our slips of the tongue, our forgetting, our prejudices, how personality is made, and many other mysteries in which we are all interested. It deals with considerable confidence in the problems of capital and labour, economic motives, peace and war. No wonder that it is attracting attention.

As we read the literature of the new psychology we stop to recall our psychological reading of ten or fifteen years

[1] Sections of this and the succeeding chapter as well as figures 2 and 3 have appeared in my article in the *Psychological Review*, vol. xxx, No. 5, September, 1923. They are reproduced here with the permission of the Editor.

ago, and we find that the two kinds of psychology do not even use the same language. The terminology is entirely different. In the psychology which has become established in universities, the categories include sensation and perception, imagination, reasoning, the sense organs, memory, the affective states, and so on. These terms have a familiar sound to anyone who has ever taken a course in psychology. In the new psychology we read about complexes, rationalization, projection, compensation, identification, symbolism, repression, the wish, and many other categories that do not even occur in the indexes of standard textbooks of the subject. What is the fundamental reason for the disparity between the established type of psychological discourse and the so-called new psychology ?

There are several factors that contribute toward this disparity in psychological language, and it is well to keep them in mind in order to understand the present tendencies in the interpretation of mental phenomena. First we must recall the different origins of the old and of the new psychology. The old psychology was written partly by philosophers and later by psychologists who devoted themselves to the scientific study of mind. The new psychology and particularly psychoanalysis has been developed by those physicians who have devoted themselves primarily to the treatment of mental disorder. Here we have two different types of training for the men who represent the two different types of psychology. In general, a fair-minded student would probably admit that the new psychology deals with subjects that are more generally interesting than those which he may recall from his textbooks. On the other hand, one must admit also that the psychology of the standard textbooks is written with greater regard for scientific consistency. The new psychology has very little regard for scientific method, and it does not rest on careful experimental work to ascertain the facts. Nevertheless, the new psychology has a strong appeal to our interests, and in large part its propositions seem to be very plausible. It is only natural that the physicians who devote themselves primarily to the treatment of disordered minds should pay attention mostly to the methods that work, while the psychologists, as scientists, should pay attention mostly to the scientific experimental methods for establishing facts.

Another factor that partly explains the difference between the new psychology and the old is to be found in the character of the mental phenomena that are the basis of the two schools. The psychiatrist deals with minds that are abnormal, minds that have broken under stress of some kind. The psychologist deals with normal minds, minds that are sufficiently calm, quiet, and contented, to submit in the psychological laboratory to experimentation. Obviously the materials on which the two schools of psychology are built up differ at the very source of the observations.

The normal person who has sufficient leisure to serve as a subject of experimentation in the psychological laboratory is not likely to have any major mental disturbance and distress. If, on the occasion of a peaceful psychological experiment, he is mentally disturbed by any serious issue in his fundamental life interests—financial, sexual, social, professional, physical—he reports that he is indisposed, and he does not serve as a subject. It is therefore relatively seldom that the psychological laboratory gets for observation persons who are in a mental condition of major significance. The psychiatrist, on the other hand, continually observes persons whose mental states are dominated, or broken, by issues that are close to the fundamental mainsprings of life.

It is only reasonable, therefore, that we should find a fundamental difference between the new and the old psychology as regards the significance of the mental phenomena that they represent. The established forms of psychological discussion relate mostly to the *momentary mental states* and related phenomena, such as the sense qualities, colour mixture, the taste buds, the visual illusions, the reflexes, peripheral vision, reaction time, the learning and forgetting of nonsense syllables, the fields of attention, visual and auditory imagery, the momentary nature of emotion, the difference between instinctive and habitual actions. All of these, and in fact most of the discussions in the standard textbooks of psychology, refer to the momentary mental states, situations in which a laboratory experiment may be prepared and in which the subject reports what he at that moment sees, or hears, or feels. There is no criticism to be made against all this scientific experimentation except that *it seldom relates to the permanent life interests* of the persons who lend their minds to the psychological experiments.

In the new psychology we deal, on the other hand, with a whole series of explanatory categories that have their origin in the psychopathic hospitals, where every person

observed is giving vent to a disturbance in the fundamental and permanent mainsprings of his life. This contrast
between the new psychology and the old is summarized
by noting that the established forms of psychological
writing deal mostly with the *momentary mental states*,
while the new psychology deals mostly with the *expression
of basic and permanent human wants*.

There are, of course, many secondary branches of these
two large schools of psychology, and there is an ever-
increasing number of men who can straddle both schools ;
but it is clear that their interest in the permanent life motives
comes from their clinical experience, while their interest
in rigorous scientific experimentation comes from the
peaceful psychological laboratory in the college.

The two schools represent two widely differing points of
view in the study of the mind, and it is our purpose in these
chapters to assist in bridging the gap so as ultimately to
combine the worthy features of both schools of thought
into a consistent interpretation of the human mind.

One of the basic differences between the old and the new
psychology is in the treatment of the stimulus or environment. Writers of the academic schools of psychology
treat the stimulus as the datum for psychological inquiry.
They put their subject into the laboratory, and confront
him with stimuli of various kinds, colours, noises, pains,
words, and with the stimulus as a starting-point they
note what happens. The behaviour of the person is
interpreted largely as a mathematical function of the
stimulus or environment. The person's own inclinations
are of course recognized as constituting a factor in the

situation, but only as a modifying factor. The stimulus is treated as the datum or starting-point, while the resulting behaviour or conduct is treated as the end-point for the psychological inquiry. The medical writers on psychology state or imply a very different interpretation of the stimulus. Here, the starting-point of conduct is the individual person himself. He wants certain things, he has cravings, desires, wishes, aspirations, ambitions, impulses. He expresses these impulses in terms of the environment. The stimulus is treated by the new psychology as only a means to an end, a means utilized by the person in getting the satisfactions that he intrinsically wants. This is a very basic contrast. In the older schools of psychology we have the characteristic sequence : the stimulus—the person— the behaviour. The behaviour is thought of mainly as replies to the stimuli. In the newer schools of psychology we have a different characteristic sequence : the person —the stimulus—the behaviour. The stimulus is treated merely as the environmental facts that we use to express our purposes.

2.   STIMULUS-RESPONSE

In the current academic psychology we teach a stimulus-response formula about which everything else psychological revolves. The contributions of the newer schools of psychology are certain to modify the rigidity of this formula. By the stimulus-response formula is meant the constant resolution of every psychological problem into three conventional parts : the *stimulus*, which is treated as a first cause, the *mind* or central nervous system, and the *behaviour*,

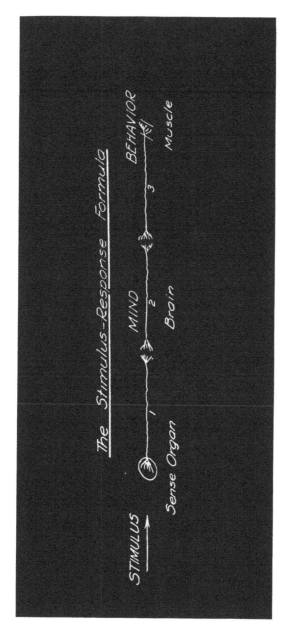

FIG. 1.

[*To face p.* 6.

which is treated as a reply to the stimulus. After some practice this formula becomes so thoroughly ingrained that every psychological question is habitually broken up into a search for the provocative stimulus, a description of the resulting mental states, and a description of the responsive behaviour.

When a mental phenomenon is to be explained, many psychologists and educators of the older schools proceed somewhat as follows. What was the stimulus? Describe it. What was the muscular response? Describe it objectively. What happened between these two things? There were " bonds " between them, and " pathways ", and " grooves " ; and " processes " took place, and there were " connexions " in the nervous system between the stimulus and the response. That settles it, and the event is psychologically explained. In order to make it clear they draw three lines on the blackboard with " fuzzy " ends to represent neurones and synapses. (See Fig. 1.) The three parts of the conventional analysis are represented diagrammatically by three neurones, one for the sense organ which receives the stimulus, one or more representing the central nervous system, and one representing the innervation of a muscle. Here we have the basic formula for psychological analysis as it is currently taught. Behaviour or conduct begins with a stimulus, and it ends with a muscular response. One cannot read the authors who represent the findings of abnormal psychology without becoming sceptical about the adequacy of this stimulus-response formula to which we have long been accustomed, although none of these writers explicitly attack the formula as such.

In Fig. 2 the two contrasting points of view are represented in a diagrammatic way. The generally current formulation is represented in the upper part of the diagram. A stimulus hits us. The mind consists of the so-called bonds and pathways, and out comes the response. When we see a muscular adjustment, we point to a known, or unknown, stimulus which has found its way transformed through bonds and pathways into our conduct. It would hardly be fair to say that we are always as totally unmindful of the mental in our mental science as the simple diagram would indicate. And yet, the great majority of discussions in psychology are carried out with this formula, either explicitly or by implication. To the student who approaches the study of psychology in expectation of discovering how his mind works, it is often a legitimate disappointment for him to learn that psychologists have reduced his mind to three unmental categories, the external physical stimulus, or the physiological stimulus, the bonds and pathways which dispose of everything mental, and the physical muscular behaviour. To relegate habitually our mental life into the unmental stimulus-response categories is a procedure which carries the appearance of science in its terminology, but which is not infrequently indicative of a superficial and unsympathetic understanding of mental life.

In the second part of Fig. 2 I have represented the function which, it seems to me, the stimulus really serves. Let us start the causal sequence with the person himself. Who and what is he ? What is he trying to do ? What kind of satisfaction is he trying to attain ? What are the types of self-expression that are especially characteristic for him ? What are the drives in him that are expressing themselves

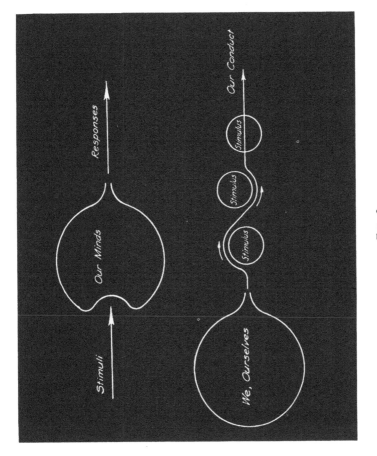

Stimuli

Our Minds

Responses

We, Ourselves

Stimulus

Stimulus

Stimulus

Our Conduct

Fig. 2.

[*To face p. 8.*

in his present conduct? Consider the stimuli as merely the environmental facts in terms of which he expresses himself. In the diagram I have represented the causal sequence as starting with the dynamic living self. Self-expression is defined into particular actions at the terminal end of the diagram. The environment, the stimulus, is causally intermediate. The stimulus determines the *detailed manner* in which a drive or purpose expresses itself on any particular occasion.

In the diagram I have attempted to show that the stimuli may be considered as of three kinds with respect to the life impulse of the organism. First, we have the stimuli that promise satisfaction of an impulse. These stimuli call forth acts of appetition. Second, we have the stimuli that mean failure. These stimuli call forth acts of aversion. Both of these types of stimuli are perceived as significant and they are determinants of conduct. Third, we have the stimuli which are entirely indifferent with respect to the impulses of the organism. These stimuli call forth no variation in conduct. If, while walking to your office in the morning, you see a coal-wagon in front of you on the sidewalk, it is a stimulus which determines an avoiding reaction. It is antagonistic to your purpose of the moment. When you see your office door in front of you it determines a positive reaction because it becomes a part of your purpose at that moment. Most of the signs, stores, vehicles, and people are indifferent stimuli which are not even perceived because you do not identify them with your purpose at the moment. In the diagram are represented two stimuli which cause avoiding reactions, and a stimulus which causes a positive reaction. The stimuli which are indifferent to the impulse or purpose are not represented in the diagram because they are not even perceived.

It is also possible to describe your actions according to the first formula. It is possible to say with accuracy that you have a visual impression of the coal-wagon, and that you respond to its presence by dodging it. The stimulus is then placed first, and your behaviour is said to be a response to the coal-wagon stimulus. The temporal sequence of such a description is correct. You first see the wagon, and then you dodge it. This is stimulus and response. It is apparent that both of these formulæ may be used with some justice to the facts. It is preferable to use the second formula because it is much more powerful as an explanatory device for complex conduct. It must be remembered that even though the stimulus precedes the response, there is usually present a purpose or objective before the appearance of the stimulus.

There are situations in which the appearance of the stimulus is sudden, and in which there cannot be said to have been any conscious purpose before the appearance of the stimulus. Such is the case when suddenly you jump out of the way in response to a Klaxon horn. You do not then have a conscious purpose to jump before the sound becomes focally conscious. The stimulus appears to be the first cause in such a situation, and it would seem to be primarily provocative of the response. It would seem to fit the first formula better, but a second consideration would bring out the fact that we are always in readiness to maintain our physical, social, financial, professional selves. To be in constant readiness to maintain, defend, and promote the self, in all its aspects, is the very essence of being alive. That is exactly the difference between an organism that is alive and one that is dead. We are so accustomed to this fundamental characteristic of every waking moment, the readiness to maintain the living self, that we do not notice it as a provocative cause for the things we do to maintain it. The Klaxon horn can then be thought of as merely the environmental circumstance at the moment by which you express that which was a part of you before the sound appeared. The sound merely determines the detailed manner in which you maintain yourself at this particular moment.

3. THE DYNAMIC SELF

In the last analysis the datum for psychology is the dynamic living self and the energy-groups into which it may be divided. We may refer to this datum as the Will to Live, or we may call it the Life-impulse, or the Vitality of the organism, or we may discover it to be the energy released by metabolism. We may be able to subdivide our will to live into large energy-groups which manifest themselves in conduct more or less independently. These energy-groups would be our innate, dynamic, and more or less distinct sources of conduct, and we might come to call them drives, motives, instincts, determining tendencies, or any other word that represents that which we as individuals innately really are, that which characterizes us as persons with individually preferred forms of life.

The living self consists of impulses to action, and the conflicts of these impulses. The conscious self I have thought of as made up of impulses that are for some reason arrested while partly formed, incomplete impulses that are in the process of becoming conduct. By this I do not mean that conscious life is different from conduct, that conscious life is merely associated with conduct by any bonds or connexions. I mean that conscious life is made of the same stuff that conduct is made of. The only difference between an idea and the corresponding action is that the idea is incomplete action. Focal consciousness consists of, is actually made of, the impulses that are in the process of becoming conduct. The aggregate of these impulses, this incomplete conduct, constitutes the momentary " me ". The permanent and more or less predictable characteristics of these impulses constitute the self. The central subject-matter of psychology is the history of these impulses from their source in the *metabolism* of the organism to their partial expressions in *thought*, to their more complete formulation in *perceived stimuli*, to their final precipitation in *overt conduct*. Conscious life is incomplete action, behaviour which is, while conscious, not sufficiently specified to constitute any definite act. Consciousness consists in impulses that are still, while conscious, too unlocalized or universal to determine anything overt. *Consciousness is the life impulse in the process of becoming conduct. To live is to telescope time.*

With our interest thus centred on the dynamic aspects of the living person himself, we are in a position of good perspective from which to study the manner in which he utilizes the stimuli of his environment, the manner in which he goes about hunting for the stimuli that the environment does not immediately give, the manner in which his dynamic self finds overt expression through and by the stimuli that happen by chance to be available, and his compromises with substitute stimuli which in other moments he would reject as inadequate. The stimulus is not primarily provocative of living, of mental life. We, ourselves, are.

4. The Psychological Act

I have just said that the central subject-matter of psychology should be the history of impulses from their source in the metabolism of the organism through the intermediate stages of formulation in which they constitute mental states, to their final expression in conduct and satisfaction to the actor. This sequence begins in the organism itself and it terminates in satisfaction to the organism itself. Between the provocative condition of the organism, which starts random or purposive behaviour, and the satisfaction which terminates the provocation of behaviour, we have all the phenomena of mind. The history, or course of events, by which a craving or want becomes neutralized in satisfaction, I shall refer to as the *psychological act*. The psychological act starts in conditions about which we know extremely little. These conditions are determined, no doubt, by the physiological state of the organism. The state of nutrition has a lot to do with it. The balance of the ductless glands is no doubt an important provocative factor in behaviour.

The psychological act is an impulse which starts in an

instinct condition. It develops into imagination by becoming more definite. It becomes still more definite when it seizes upon a sense impression as part of its own attributes. It defines itself completely when it issues in final overt form as action.

In Fig. 2 we have the psychological act divided, tentatively, into three phases: (1) the dynamic self as the origin of impulses that constitute living ; (2) the mental phase of these impulses in which they have taken some degree of definition or form ; and (3) the overt phase at which they have completed themselves in action. An overt act, the seen behaviour, is the terminal end of a psychological act. The latter consists not only of the seen conduct but also of the mental and physiological antecedents of conduct.

5. PSYCHOLOGY AS A SCIENCE

Every scientific problem is a search for the functional relation between two or more variables. This can be seen very clearly in the exact sciences, but it becomes more obscure as we enter the biological sciences, and it is frequently lost sight of in the social sciences. In physics we have, as typical problems, the search for relation between the length of time that a body has been falling and its speed, the pressure of a gas and its temperature or volume, the curvature of a lens and its focal distance, the resistance of a wire as determined by its cross-section or length, the pressure on a turbine as determined by the head in the penstock, the sag of a beam as determined by the load and the cross-section of the beam. Physicists and engineers come to look upon the search for relations between variables as the typical task of science. The attitude of looking for these relations becomes second nature to them. They reach habitually for a piece of cross-section paper in order to make a graph of the observations, and in order to visualize the nature of the relation that they are seeking.

In the biological sciences we have the same logic in the biometric methods. In the social sciences we are dealing, usually, with variables that are not quantitative, but there is no good reason why thinking in the social sciences should not follow the same logic even though the variables are often non-quantitative.

If every scientific problem is an attempt to state the relation between two or more variables, it should be profitable to note what the variables are that constitute scientific psychology. If we look over the field of experimental psychology, as it is represented by standard textbooks in the field, and by the work in psychological laboratories, we find that the relations into which the experimenters inquire classify themselves mostly in the following types :—

(1) Relation between anatomy of the sense-organs and conscious sense-experience. Typical for such experiments are the studies to determine the relation between the touch, cold, and heat spots in the skin and the corresponding cutaneous sensations, or the sense qualities of colour that we have in the different parts of the retina. Another example would be the relation between the parts of the internal ear and sense-experience.

(2) Relation between stimuli and sense-experience. Here we have such typical laboratory experiments as the

determination of the laws of colour mixture. The relation studied is that between the description of the colours that are being mixed and the sense-experience which is the result.

(3) Relation between stimuli and muscular adjustment. The reaction time experiments are typical of this class. The reaction time experiment is an attempt to predict behaviour in terms of the conditions of the stimuli which are arranged as the cue for the behaviour.

Totally different is the fundamental nature of the relations that the medical writers in psychology are dealing with. They are constantly searching for the relation between the fundamental cravings and wants of people and the ways in which these wants are expressed. A patient talks and behaves as though he were an emperor, a millionaire, a person with power and fame. Let us contrast the two different scientific approaches of the old and the new psychology to this problem. What are the variables involved in the problem ? The psychologist of the established academic schools would ask about the stimuli, the environment, and he would state or imply in his solution that the patient is merely responding to stimuli. There might be some difficulty in specifying just what the stimuli are to which the patient is responding by talking like an emperor. The academic psychologist would list on one side of his scientific ledger the stimuli and environment to which the patient has been exposed, and on the other side of the ledger would be recorded the behaviour of the patient. The conduct would be described as a function of the environment, modified, to be sure, by the characteristics of the patient himself.

The psychiatrist would look for a different set of variables. He would list on one side of his ledger the wants and cravings of normal people, assuming that these wants are also part of the self of the patient, and on the other side of the ledger he would list the patient's conduct. The scientific problem would be to state how it comes about that the patient expresses in his particular way wants that are universal. The psychiatrist would treat the environment as merely the means by which the patient seeks to express wants and cravings that are universal. This procedure is much more powerful and illuminating. It shows us more about human nature, but it is not subject to the exact quantitative technique of the older sciences because the wants and cravings of normal people have not yet been classified and isolated in a measurable way.

Let us consider a typical laboratory experiment as another illustration. I have said that we are in the habit of describing action as a function of the stimulus. We place before a subject a tachistoscope, and he sees nonsense syllables. He tries over and over again until he has learned them. Out of this psychological experiment comes the scientific deduction that, other things being equal, he remembers best those syllables which are at the end of the list and which he saw last. He tends to remember also quite well those syllables that he saw first, before the novelty wore off. He does not remember so well the syllables in the middle of the list. This is a scientific experiment in which we state the relationship between two variables. The answers of the subject are described as a function of the stimulating nonsense. But how about incentives ?   The most important factor is whether or not he cares about the nonsense syllables.   This factor of interest and effort overshadows entirely the small effects of the arrangement of the syllables.   The experiment is scientifically quite legitimate, but it is trivial in respect to the factors that are most important for mental life.

We recognize, of course, this fact, that incentives are more important than the arrangement of the syllables on the page in predicting the recall.   But since the incentives are not readily measured, we rest content with describing the relations that we *can* measure.   Well and good.   This would not be subject to criticism if it were not for the fact that we have come to forget the individual person altogether. Experiments of this type have come to be the rule, and we have taken for granted that psychology is primarily concerned with the incidental relation between the response and the response-modifying stimulus.   We have gone so far as to assert that psychology studies the stimulus-response relation, and we have forgotten the person himself who may or may not want to do the responding.

I suggest that we dethrone the stimulus.   He is only nominally the ruler of psychology.   The real ruler of the domain which psychology studies is the individual and his motives, desires, wants, ambitions, cravings, aspirations. The stimulus is merely the more or less accidental fact in the environment, and it becomes a stimulus only when it serves as a tool for somebody's purposes.   When it does not serve as a tool for getting us what we want, it is no longer a stimulus.   It is not a cause.   It is simply a means by which we achieve our own ends, not those of

THE STIMULUS-RESPONSE FORMULA

The stimulus————————Human wants————————The response

THE SELF-EXPRESSION FORMULA

Human wants————————The stimulus————————Conduct

Fig. 3.

[To face p. 18.

the stimulus. The psychological act which is the central subject-matter of psychology becomes then the course of events, primarily mental, which intervene between the motive and the successful neutralization or satisfaction of that motive. The stimulus appears somewhere between the provocative and the overt terminals of the psychological act. Mental life consists primarily in the approximate formulation of the motives leading toward overt expression. To the extent that mental life is of a relatively high order these approximate formulations of the motives become more and more tentative, deliberate, inhibited, delayed, and subject to choice before precipitating into their final overt form.

This point of view that I am recommending is not so radical as it might at first sight appear. What I am recommending is after all merely a shift of emphasis diagrammatically represented in Fig. 3. In that figure the upper line represents the causal chain tacitly followed by psychology as it is now usually written. This chain of events starts with the stimulus as the fundamental datum for psychological inquiry. From the stimulus as a source we trace the mental events to the response. Between these two terminals we place the characteristics of the individual in the form of modifying mental sets, predispositions, irritability, instincts, habits. We admit that the individual does enter into the causal chain but only as a modifier of the stimulus-response series. When we talk about instincts, for example, we look first of all for a suitable stimulus which can be given the credit for starting the instinctive behaviour. The stimulus is assumed to be the absolutely essential starting-point for an instinctive act. At the other end of the causal chain we set down the characteristic behaviour which is brought about by the particular stimulus. Between these two events we assume that the individual himself has something to say but only as a modifier of the fundamental stimulus-response relation.

In the second line of Fig. 3, I have represented the individual and the stimulus as exchanging their places. The individual is in this second representation assumed to be the starting-point for that which he himself does. The stimulus takes the secondary rôle of modifier. The primary formula is then to be found in the impulse-conduct relation. The expression of the impulse is of course markedly affected by the stimuli, which are now to be considered as the momentary circumstances of the environment. I am simply shifting the stimulus to the secondary rôle of a modifier, and I am promoting the individual and his life impulses to the first rank of cause as far as psychology is concerned.

Consider the instinctive adjustments of retaliation against an insult. The insult would be described as a stimulus. Your defence would be described as a response. If you have lately been on the defensive as regards your position, professional status, financial security, or health, your motive of self-defence or self-preservation would have a low threshold. A trivial remark from an insignificant source might be sufficient to arouse defensive conduct on your part such as a fist blow, loss of temper, loud, self-assertive talk, sullenness, or a domineering manner towards associates. If you have lately enjoyed a feeling of relative security with reference to your social, professional, financial, and physical self, the threshold for this defensive behaviour would be so high that the trivial remark would be passed unnoticed.

If you do reply to it, one would, of course, say that the insulting remarks came first, and that your reply came afterward. But such a stimulus-response analysis of the situation would be superficial. It would not be the remark that drove you on to defend yourself. The stimulus is only an environmental fact which determines partly how you express your desire at the moment. It is psychologically much more interesting to discover the tendencies that seek expression than to describe conduct as merely replies to stimuli.

Suppose that you are stuck on a country road on account of an engine which has been maltreated. There were surely stimuli that preceded your inspection of the engine. That which makes you do things to that engine is not primarily the stimuli from the engine—it is your desire to go. The stimuli are simply environmental facts which modify the expression of your desire to get there.

It may well be that our stimulus-response habits in psychological discussion came about because of the obvious fact that the stimulus often precedes conscious solution, and this in turn often precedes the overt act. The insulting remark no doubt preceded your back-talk, the engine balked before you looked for the trouble. That is all true, but your unsatisfied desire for security was active as an unlocalized irritability before the insulting remark was made, and your desire to keep on going was being actively satisfied before the engine balked. The facts of temporal sequence should not blind us to the major causal factors of mental life.

6. Stimulus-response in the Animal Mind

This point of view is not limited to the interpretation of the human mind. It applies as well to the behaviour of the lower organisms. We are too often inclined to look upon the animal mind as consisting of nothing but reflexes acting in response to the stimuli that happen to strike it.

Let me quote from Jennings.[1] " Activity does not require present external stimulation. A first and essential point for the understanding of behaviour is that activity occurs in organisms without present specific external stimulation. The normal condition of Paramecium is an active one, with its cilia in rapid motion ; it is only under special conditions that it can be brought partly to rest. Vorticella, as Hodge and Aikins showed, is at all times active, never resting. The same is true of most other infusoria, and, in perhaps a less marked degree, of many other organisms. Even if external movements are suspended at times, internal activities continue. The *organism is activity,* and its activities may be spontaneous, so far as present external stimuli are concerned. . . . The spontaneous activity, of course, depends finally on external conditions, in the same sense that the existence of the organism depends on external conditions. Reaction by selection of excess movements depends largely

---

[1] Jennings, H. S., *Behaviour of the Lower Organisms,* chaps. 16, 18.

on the fact that the movement itself is not directly produced by the stimulus. The movement is due, as we have seen, to the internal energy of the organism. . . . The energy for the motion comes from within and is merely released by the action of the stimulus. It is important to remember, if the behaviour is to be understood, that energy, and often impulse to movement, comes from within, and that when they are released by the stimulus, this is merely what James has called ' trigger action '."

I will of course admit that the life-impulses depend on the environment. So does the very life of the organism. The life-impulse is derived from the metabolism of the organism, and this is in turn contingent on what the environment gives. That is all true. But I should insist that psychology begin with the life-impulse as its datum, and that it be concerned with the mental routes by which the impulse expresses itself.

The life-impulse has a history leading back to past stimuli, but the sequence from these stimuli to the accretion of vitality is a biological rather than a psychological problem. Except for some division of the task, one could readily find oneself arguing in a circle as to what it is that starts the whole business, the life-impulse or the stimulus. Mental life is an irreversible process beginning with the life-impulse and terminating in the successful overt act. The stimulus may be thought of as a means for specifying the approximate act which is mental. Present overt action, and the approximate actions which constitute mental life, can only very roughly be stated in terms of the individual's stimulus-history.

CHAPTER II

THE CLASSIFICATION OF BEHAVIOUR

1. *Antecedents and consequences of action*
2. *Stages of the psychological act*
   (a) *Energy-source*
   (b) *Lowered threshold for stimuli*
   (c) *Deliberate ideation*
   (d) *The internal stimulus*
   (e) *Imaginal hunt for external stimuli*
   (f) *Overt hunt for external stimuli*
   (g) *The external stimulus*
   (h) *The consummatory overt act*
   (i) *Overt consequences of the act*
   (k) *Satisfaction to the actor and quiescence at the energy-source*

1. ANTECEDENTS AND CONSEQUENCES OF ACTION

One of the basic problems in psychology is necessarily the classification of actions and their incomplete forms which constitute conscious life. There are different bases by which actions may be classified. The simplest of these is that of direct similarity of the overt acts themselves. To pick up a fork, and to pick up a fountain-pen, are two acts that are closely similar, and they may for certain narrow purposes be classified together. Psychologically two such actions are totally different in two respects. The mental antecedents of the two overt acts are totally different, and the consequences and immediate satisfactions are also different. If we compare the two psychological acts that are involved we find that they converge at one point only, namely at the point where the motives or purposes issue into overt expressions. Before and after this point the two acts and their consequences cannot be classified together. From the standpoint of the psychologist it is a negligible circumstance that the two psychological acts happen to terminate in the same muscle groups.

We may proceed in either direction, through the antecedents or through the consequences of the act, in order to discover other bases for classifying action. Let us go to the antecedents first. If two psychological acts are similar in the mental antecedents of the overt acts, the two resulting actions may for that reason be classified together. Suppose you discover that you should have given some information to another man. This is a mental state and it is therefore unfinished action. The resulting overt formulation of the psychological act may take various forms. You may reach for the telephone, or you may put on your hat and coat and walk out. These two seen forms of behaviour are, of course, different in appearance, but there was a point in the mental antecedents of two such possible actions at which they would be identical, namely that stage in the formulation of behaviour which is merely the realization that some information should be conveyed. Two widely different overt acts may, then, have converged, and they may have been identical, at some mental antecedent stage. We see that if we define the psychological act as the *whole course* of events from a purpose or motive, through its imaginal form, through the overt expression, to the consequences and satisfactions to the actor, we have numerous points at which different psychological acts may be treated as identical even though they differ widely at other stages.

Two acts may be declared to be in the same category because of the fact that they converge and are identical at the point where the stimulus appears. The stimulus for the *exteroceptors*[1] constitutes a relatively late and rather completely formulated phase of the psychological act. The stimulus for the *interoceptors*[2] constitutes an earlier and less definitely formulated phase of behaviour. It often happens that a stimulus for the interoceptors is the first conscious presence of the unfinished behaviour which completes itself in a hunt for suitable stimulation of the exteroceptors. These latter stimuli in turn complete themselves as ordinary percepts into overt action and resulting satisfaction, or into a continued hunt for more stimuli. Two psychological acts may be declared to belong in the same category because of the similarity of the internal or external stimuli by which the several lines of unfinished behaviour converge or are identical.

A more important and fundamental basis of classification would be the possible identity of several types of behaviour at their energy-source. It may be possible to discover that the total energy of the organism, which is derived from its

---

[1] An exteroceptor is a sense-organ excited by stimuli outside the body.
[2] An interoceptor is a sense-organ excited by stimuli arising within the viscera.

metabolism, is divisible into energy-groups. It is not impossible to imagine that in one organism much of the energy may turn to digestive functions with resulting keen interest and satisfaction in food. In another organism a relatively smaller proportion of the energy which it accumulates is turned into this direction. There may well be individual differences in the division of the total energy of the organism into the several groups which constitute the source of its life-impulses. In a similar manner organisms of the same species may differ in the relative proportion of their total energy which normally goes into the sex functions. In the human it is also conceivable that there are individual differences in the proportions of energy which normally seek expression in aggressive and self-assertive behaviour, in sex life, in digestion, in locomotion, in gregarious conduct, and so on. It may well be that the different behaviour of the prize-fighter and the scholar converge as identical in that early phase of their conduct in which both seek social approval. Both may be so absorbed in the immediate detail of what they are doing that they do not consciously realize the identity of the source of their labours.

It is in these energy-sources of conduct that we shall find the distinctions between instincts. Instincts can never be defined in terms of the stimuli by which we happen to express ourselves ; nor can they ever be defined in terms of particular behaviour on particular occasions. The futility of the instinct category in psychology inheres in the fact that we have been looking for a specific stimulus on which to attach a specific instinctive response. The only point in the great variety of behaviour at which the psychological acts belonging to an instinct are identical is at the energy-source.

If, instead of proceeding from the overt act toward the mental and the unconscious antecedents, we follow the psychological acts into their consequences, we find still additional points at which they may converge. Two psychological acts may be totally different, but they may conceivably have similar immediate consequences as objectively determined. Such a fact would be a legitimate basis of classification.

Still another basis for classifying actions together would be in the degree to which they may be substituted for each other with equal satisfaction to the actor. This is one of the most useful explanatory devices in psychology.

2. STAGES OF THE PSYCHOLOGICAL ACT

I have listed a number of stages in the development of psychological acts in which they may be identical or similar. If we start with action at its source and follow the stages through which it becomes formulated into conduct, and the consequent satisfactions, we shall have a table as follows :—

(a) Energy-source
(b) Lowered threshold for stimuli
(c) Deliberate ideation
(d) The internal stimulus
(e) Imaginal hunt for external stimuli
(f) Overt hunt for external stimuli

(g) The external stimulus
(h) The consummatory overt act
(i) Overt consequences of the act
(k) Satisfaction to the actor and quiescence at the energy-source

The energy-source.—The sources of conduct are the physiological, mental, and social conditions of satiety or satisfaction which every normal person seeks. These physical and mental conditions cover such categories as the satisfaction of hunger, bodily comfort, sex, social approval, social power. A state of dissatisfaction in any one of the instinct conditions is the starting-point for action which is maintained until satisfaction is attained. Two actions belong in the same instinct category if they may, by conditioning, be readily substituted. Two actions belong in different instinct categories if they can only, by prolonged conditioning, be substituted for each other. It may be that the instinct sources of behaviour are not truly energy-groups, but only physiological and mental conditions which make demands on the total energy-supply of the organism for random or purposive behaviour until conditions of satisfaction are attained.

Lowered threshold for stimuli.—When an instinct condition is in a state of dissatisfaction there results a lowered threshold for relevant stimuli long before the appearance of conscious need, desire, or purpose. At five o'clock in the afternoon we are normally more easily tempted by the smell of a good steak than immediately after lunch, but in the absence of the external stimulus we may be entirely unaware of the lowered sensory and interest threshold. The instinct condition has by its lowered threshold already started to determine the ultimate behaviour before any conscious or external indices appear. The behaviour is already on its course of formulation before the internal or external stimulus appears.

Deliberate ideation.—In the instinct condition of a dissatisfaction which has not yet become sufficiently acute to be conscious in sensory form, and in which the actor is not himself aware of the lowered interest threshold, the expected behaviour appears in imaginal form. Biologically the purpose of ideation is to prepare for action. The actor himself may not be aware of the fact that his thinking has its source in some state of incompleteness or dissatisfaction in the physical or social self. Since the need is not urgent or explicitly conscious, the actor's thinking is correspondingly calm and deliberate.

The internal stimulus is parallel to the stage of deliberate ideation in the formulation of behaviour, but it represents in those instinct conditions, where it normally takes part, a more definitely specified form of the behaviour than the ideation which precedes or accompanies it.

Imaginal hunt for the external stimulus represents a later and more complete formulation of behaviour than the free-moving, purposeless thought, and its relatives in internal stimuli. At this stage of the definition of conduct we have the expected experience in conscious form, and it has taken sufficient definition to be introspectively recognized as purposive. It is in reality an imaginal hunt for those suitable environmental stimuli which, if found, lead to consummatory action. It is purposive imaginal preparation for expected experience. Expected conduct is now beginning to take sufficient cognitive form to be the subject of imaginal trial-and-error choice. This is realistic thinking which is purposive as contrasted with autistic thinking, which is less definitely purposive. Both forms of thinking are driven by instinct conditions.

Overt hunt for external stimuli is merely carrying the purposive thinking into action in the hope of finding the imaginally expected stimuli. These overt actions may be directed immediately toward the significant stimulus, or they may be random in the nature of overt trial and error. It happens not infrequently that an instinct condition leads to overt random search without any conscious purpose, and without any definite conscious realization of the nature of the satisfaction that is sought.

The external stimulus represents a rather late stage in the formulation of behaviour. The psychological act is almost completed at the appearance of the external stimulus. The meaning of the stimulus is the expected satisfaction of the instinct condition for which the organism is ready. Many of the external stimuli are consciously sought, hunted for. The external stimuli which appear suddenly, such as danger signals, have as their meaning the maintenance of bodily integrity, a condition which by the mere fact of living, the organism is in constant readiness to maintain.

The consummatory overt act is the terminal of what I have called the psychological act.

The overt consequences of the act are in most cases practically parallel with the consummatory act and with the satisfactions to the actor.

The satisfaction to the actor consists in quiescence at the energy-source. It should be noted that the beginning of this sequence and the end of it are identical in character. Behaviour starts in the instinct condition, and it terminates in the satisfied instinct condition. It is in this sense that we can speak of a reflex circuit rather than the reflex arc. We have traced the psychological sequence by which behaviour is formed. The mental antecedents of behaviour constitute in fact behaviour in the process of being particularized.

CHAPTER III

MIND AS UNFINISHED CONDUCT

1. STATEMENT OF THE PRINCIPLE

My main thesis is that consciousness is unfinished action. This idea is by no means novel because all psychological discussion of thinking, emotion, and the will, assumes that there is a normal issue in conduct of mental processes. To reason is, of course, normally to reason about something and that something has its final verification in action. To be in an emotional state always implies action, or the inhibition of action, or the frustrating of intended action. Emotion can hardly be thought of as existing in the absence of implied action. Similarly with the volitional states which are by definition directly related to action, or its inhibition. Therefore, to say that consciousness is unfinished action is in harmony with all schools of psychology, but the blunt statement that every mental state is an unfinished act is, at least in this phrasing, rather uncommon.

Exception might be taken to the assertion that consciousness is, fundamentally, action that is in the process of being formed, by pointing to the sense-impressions and to free imagery. We can imagine a flight of colours and shapes without any very definite intention to carry the imagery into action. This is true, as far as definite intentions towards overt action are concerned, but, normally, imagery does not appear except as part of a conscious or sub-conscious want. Most of our thoughts during the course of a day are in definite relation to the things that we expect to do overtly in some form. I hope to show in the following chapters that every mental state is, fundamentally, unfinished action, even though we are not always fully aware of any definite intention to carry the mental state into an immediate act.[1]

Closely related to our proposition that mental states are unfinished acts is the psychological phenomenon known as ideo-motor action. By this term is meant the close connexion that is sometimes seen between an idea and its equivalent immediate fulfilment in overt form. Technically defined, ideo-motor action is the expression of an idea into muscular form without further conscious deliberation or hesitancy. Whenever there is a conflict between the idea, considered as an unfinished act, and another idea, there is delay or inhibition in the execution, and the sequence is not then termed ideo-motor action in the strict sense. The basic relation, when there is no conflict or deliberation, is that of an idea which issues forthwith into the action

---

[1] See Chapter IX for a discussion of the sense-qualities in relation to this principle.

that corresponds with the idea.   In his discussion of this subject James says: " Consciousness is *in its very nature impulsive* " (his own italics).   Most of our habitual actions, tipping the hat, turning a familiar corner, grasping the telephone receiver, are carried out without conflict or conscious intent.   The mere presence of the idea is enough, and the idea completes itself by becoming action.   It is only when there is a conflict between two unfinished or proposed actions, two conflicting ideas, that the effect of ideo-motor action is withheld.   We shall see that if we consider this ideo-motor tendency, not as a special psychological phenomenon, but as a universal tendency for all conscious life, the resulting interpretation of the several cognitive categories in psychology takes a form somewhat different from the conventional definitions.

In the preceding section I have declared that our minds are not primarily actuated by the stimuli of the environment, but that mind is better thought of as the intermediary between the instinct conditions and the behaviour by which the instinct conditions are neutralized.   We have, then, a sequence of three phases, starting with the conditions of bodily and mental dissatisfactions, that we do not recognize introspectively at their source.   These instinct conditions that constitute the prime movers of behaviour are partly physical, such as the maintenance of bodily comfort, freedom from hunger, and sex satisfaction, and partly mental, such as the maintenance of social approval, and self-advancement.   An instinct condition which is in a state of relative satisfaction figures correspondingly less in determining what the organism thinks and struggles for, except for the situation in which one satisfied instinct condition is over-emphasized to compensate for another instinct condition which is failing of satisfaction.

The second phase of the circuit is conscious life proper, in which the wants and the aspirations that originate as instinct conditions have taken some tentative form of expected adjustment. To think is to expect to act. To think is also necessarily to entertain a conflict between two or more acts. Except for the conflict there would be no thought. The thought would forthwith become action. The third phase of the circuit is behaviour itself.

The three phases of the circuit, the instinct conditions that constitute the momentary self, the tentative formulations of the momentary self toward expected behaviour, and the behaviour itself, are all made of the same stuff. The circuit should not be thought of as made up of three compartments with definable separating walls. The instinct condition becomes with increased definition and specification the mental state, and this in turn becomes, by increased particulars, the overt conduct. The psychological act is just this sequence from the vague state of want through the approximate formulations of action which constitute mental life in the functional sense, to the completely formulated action which is the muscular activity itself.

The psychological act represents an energy translation from a state in which it is diffuse, not consciously localized, universal, toward a state in which it is closely specified as the energy of movement. There is, however, a fundamental difference between the translation represented by the three phases of the reflex circuit, and the translation with which we are familiar in the passage of energy through a machine. If we want to study a complicated machine, we start, logically, with the entry of energy into the machine, and we follow the energy through pulleys and gears until we arrive at the terminal, in a cutting edge perhaps. The localization of energy may be as definite at the power drive of the machine as it is at the cutting edge. It is different with the energy translation through the reflex circuit. We cannot profitably start at the energy-source with our present limited knowledge in the biological sciences. We can, however, start at the terminal or behaviour end of the circuit, for this is definite and observable. We can trace the antecedents of the behaviour through at least some of its preceding forms as purposes and wants, and we can under certain circumstances see how mental states represent desired objective ends even when the actor himself is not aware of the aim that he is really trying to attain. Work in the abnormal field amply illustrates how mental life is determined in its course by ends which the actor or thinker is not himself aware of, but which must have a source in some unsatisfied instinct condition in the actor.

We can start, then, with a close description of behaviour or conduct, and it should be our aim to find the antecedents of behaviour in the mental life of the actor. Now, it so happens that the farther we go from overt behaviour through the mental antecedents toward the instinct sources of conduct, the more vague, unlocalized, tentative, and universal is the form of the psychological act. If we push our inquiry far into the mental antecedents of behaviour we come, sooner or later, to those stages in the formulation of behaviour in which the expected conduct has not taken sufficiently definite shape to be recognizable as a particular form of behaviour. The act is in those early phases so loosely organized that it is impossible to equate it with certainty to any particular overt act through which it may finally express itself. The final behaviour by which instinct conditions are neutralized is the centre of reference about which psychological inquiry should radiate. It is the behaviour which successfully neutralizes instinctive wants that the organism thinks toward, and our interpretation of conscious life should be in terms of the expected successful behaviour for which mental processes are only tentative preparations. The main idea is that we are first of all living beings, and only in a secondary sense reactors to our environment. If our impulses to live are denied their satisfying expression by some limitation in the environment, we either hunt restlessly about until agreeable stimuli are found, or we identify ourselves with substitute stimuli that we would ignore in a more favourable environment.

If you have been walking in the country for hours without companionship, it is not at all unnatural to find yourself interested in the first stranger you meet. In your customary environment you may have limited your companionship to those of your own kind, ignoring those who differ from you markedly. To say that the stranger is a stimulus to whom you respond as a reactor is to lose the psychologically most important aspect of the situation, namely, your impulse and readiness to be social.

The nature of the translation that takes place in the reflex circuit can be illustrated by the terms *extension* and *intension*. The instinct condition which originates conduct has a maximum of extension, a minimum of intension. By this is meant that the condition can find final expression in almost any number of different forms of behaviour which are not yet specified. It is a universal of the highest order. As the condition translates itself into the mentally expected adjustment it becomes slightly more specified, its extension is decreased, its intension is increased by the accretion of attributes. The final expression of the want into overt behaviour is a condition representing a minimum of extension because it now applies only to one particular muscular adjustment at the particular moment when it is made, and it is simultaneously represented by an increase in intension because its attributes are all specified. It is this fundamental characteristic of the translation through the stages of the reflex circuit that makes it difficult to start psychological inquiry at the beginning of the sequence. We are then dealing with universals, bodily or mental. It may, of course, ultimately, be possible to identify these psychological universals as specific bodily forms, but such a discovery would be a physiological rather than a psychological contribution.

I have said that conscious life is intermediate between our impulses to live and our conduct, and that the process is essentially irreversible. The function that consciousness serves is to make our life-impulses profitable in a biological sense. *It is probable that consciousness would never have appeared except for the fact that it has survival value.* Such value it can have only in so far as it prepares action. The forward-looking function of consciousness is its reason for existence. Retrospection, memory, cannot have any value whatever except as an aid to the more fundamental forward-looking function of conscious life. Conscious life is in fact expected adjustment in the process of being formed. It is in this sense that we can say that the process is an irreversible one, beginning with the impulses that constitute life, consisting in the second phase of the tentative formulations of these impulses that constitute mental life, and completing itself in the expressions of these same impulses that constitute conduct.

If we declare an identity to exist throughout this irreversible sequence it is of course interesting to inquire as to the basis for differentiating its successive phases. *The most fundamental basis on which to differentiate the early and the late phases of the psychological act is in the degree of definition and completeness that it has at any moment attained.*

The different cognitive categories can best be recognized on this basis. A percept is a psychological act that is almost complete. It is *almost* an overt act, whereas a concept is a psychological act that is still vague and loosely formed.

If I perceive a puddle on the sidewalk in front of me the percept is a psychological act which is nearly defined. It is still subject to some further definition, because I may turn to the right, step out on the curb, jump over the puddle, or step into it. If there were no further definition possible the act would not become conscious even at its perceptual stage of completion. Consciousness, functionally considered, is the state of hesitancy at which further particulars must be supplied in order to complete the psychological act into overt form. A psychological act that is almost ready to precipitate into action is a percept.

Imagination is a psychological act which is still less defined than the percept. If you are telling me that a certain restaurant is better than the one at which we have been eating, the imaginal terms in which I participate in the conversation constitute a psychological act which is, at its imaginal stage, less defined than if I were standing across the street, looking at that restaurant. If you are telling me how to construct the supports for some shelves, my imagination is unfinished action. You may tell me to cut a notch here—on a drawing. When I understand you, I am imagining that notch, but I have not defined at this imaginal stage of the act just how I shall cut the notch, how I shall hold the boards with my hands, or the tools I shall use. These are further specifications of the act which are not necessarily present at the imaginal stage. There is no sharp line of demarcation between the perceptual and imaginal stages of the psychological act beyond the criterion of perceptual presence of some of the data. The meaning of a percept is imaginal, and in this way the two categories are continuous.

The concept is a psychological act which is very loosely defined. My concept "typewriter" is a psychological act, so incomplete that all I know is that my adjustment will be concerned somehow with a typewriter. The concept stage of the act does not even specify whether it is my typewriter that we are talking about, whether it is to be moved to another desk, whether I shall write on it, or you borrow it, or something else. The concept does not contain enough to specify any of these. Normally, however, the concept implies a readiness to do something about a typewriter. The imaginal and perceptual stages of the act define it more closely until the act is completely specified in overt form.

The customary textbook treatment of the concept gives the student the impression that the concept is a retrospective affair—a something that is common to many of his past experiences. One must have seen several dogs in order to have a concept " dog ". This is true. The concept " dog " is that which is common to all the dogs that we have met in our past experience. This is also true. This tells us how the concept is *formed*, but it does not tell us what the concept *is* when it actually appears in our daily thinking. *When the concept appears normally in our daily life it is an unfinished act which points toward a type of adjustment, an adjustment which has not yet been closely defined.* The retrospective derivation of the concept is an interesting but secondary matter.[1]

The different cognitive categories represent primarily different degrees of completion of the psychological act. The lower perceptual categories are acts which are almost ready to precipitate in overt form. The higher cognitive categories such as ideation and conception are unfinished

---

[1] Thurstone, L. L., " The anticipatory aspect of consciousness ": *Journal of Philosophy, Psychology, and Scientific Method*, vol. xvi, No. 21, 9th October, 1919.

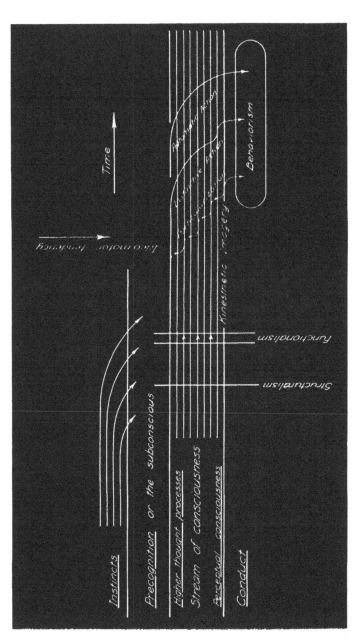

Fig. 4.

[*To face p. 42.*

acts which are as yet only loosely formed and which need further definition before they can issue in overt form.

A desire is an act in its early stage of definition. As it defines itself through conceptual thinking toward perceptual and overt form, it increases its intension and decreases its extension. When it issues in overt expression, it has all its characteristics defined and has therefore its maximum intension. At this stage it has also reduced its extension attributes since it applies only to one particular occasion. The concept is a psychological act which has a minimum of intension and correspondingly a maximum of extension, because it may issue into any one of many particular forms. The higher the concept, the fewer will be the attributes it contains and the greater will be the number of situations into which it may define itself.

2. THE STRUCTURAL INTERPRETATION OF MIND

I shall refer to the diagrammatic representation in Fig. 4. The horizontal lines in this diagram represent the stream of consciousness. Time is indicated by the arrow pointing to the right. Any vertical line or plane across the horizontal lines will therefore represent a moment of time. Any other vertical line drawn further to the right will indicate a later moment of time. The instinctive sources of action are indicated at the upper part of the diagram, and overt expression is indicated at the lower part of the diagram. The arrows pointing downward represent the fact that the instincts tend to express themselves in action. The fact that these arrows cross the stream of consciousness represents the fact that consciousness is an intermediary between the instinctive sources and overt adjustment. If an arrow be drawn on this diagram so as to point down with a steep angle, we should be representing an instinct which expresses itself suddenly without much conscious participation and within a short space of time. If another line be drawn pointing downward with a more gentle slope we should be representing an instinct which expresses itself with more conscious participation and with delayed expression into overt form.

The structural point of view in psychology is represented by the vertical line which is so labelled. By this I want to show that the structuralist is primarily interested in the momentary psychosis.[1] He attempts to catch each moment as it flies and describes it afterwards as best he can. He becomes very expert at doing this. He wants to know what is contained in the momentary mental state. He finds elements in it which he classifies and names. His system is a method of describing and classifying as completely as possible the momentary cross-section of the stream of consciousness. He is not especially interested in the fact that there is a stream, that there is action with time. Of course he does not deny it, but his main interest is to discover the elements in the momentary mental states. He puts them together and arranges a system very much as a chemist might arrange and classify elements. One of his main jobs is to describe from memory as completely as possible everything that was in his mind at any one moment of time.

[1] A psychosis is any mental state, any moment of consciousness.

3. THE FUNCTIONAL INTERPRETATION OF MIND

Having gone far in the description and classification of various psychoses it was only natural that one should turn one's attention to the question as to how the mind works. This point of view in psychology is called functional. The emphasis here is on the stream of consciousness, its shifts from one psychosis to another—the resolution of the psychosis. Having described the elements of a momentary psychosis with the structural interest, we turn to ask what becomes of them, thus changing to a functional interest. This slightly different attitude necessitates the modification of some fundamental definitions. Instead of describing the momentary psychoses as such, we describe them with more reference to what they tend to become. This point of view appeals to the student more readily than the structural point of view because it has more dynamic interest. It is of more human interest to inquire how a thing works than to possess a complete description and classification of that thing at rest.

The functional point of view is represented in the diagram as a section of the stream of consciousness between two vertical lines that are fairly close together. I have placed several small arrows within this range to show that the functional point of view recognizes that consciousness is dynamic.[1] The functionalist in psychology is interested in the character of the processes that go on in consciousness, but he confines himself to these with a very limited range in time.

[1] The fact that functionalism is diagrammatically to the right of structuralism is only a matter of graphical convenience and is not intended to have any interpretation.

4. THE BEHAVIOURISTIC INTERPRETATION OF MIND

The general plan of the diagram is intended to show that the biological purpose of consciousness is to mediate action. Consciousness owes its existence to the fact that it has made our adjustments more effective. It is interesting to note that if the three points of view which are represented in the diagram are arranged in the historical order in which they appeared, we have an increasing emphasis on the dynamic significance of consciousness. The structuralist is interested primarily in discovering what the momentary mental state really is. The functionalist is more interested in discovering how the momentary mental state shifts and resolves. The behaviourist is primarily interested in behaviour itself. In fact, he is so interested in overt behaviour that he forgets its conscious antecedents altogether.

In the diagram I have represented the behaviouristic point of view as limited to the behaviour into which mental life normally issues. One objects to the behaviouristic emphasis on overt behaviour to the exclusion of the antecedent mental states. To follow such a point of view would mean the exclusion of mental life from the content of psychology, and that we should hardly be willing to allow. But there is something fundamentally sound in the behaviouristic interest in overt adjustment. Consciousness exists in order to serve overt adjustment. We should therefore study mental life with overt behaviour as our central explanatory base.

My point of view is in a sense a cross between function-alism and behaviourism. I am interested in the stream of consciousness, but my interpretation of it is entirely guided by the overt adjustments into which it issues. I shall be inclined to classify together those mental elements which serve the same type of overt adjustment, or the same type of biological purpose, even if the several mental elements are seemingly disparate. Such a procedure should be fruitful because we shall then be guided by the functions which the mental elements serve rather than by their appear-ance in the momentary state. Studies in behaviourism are of value to psychology only in so far as they throw light on the conscious antecedents. The study of behaviourism is in psychology only a means to an end, and not an end in itself. Behaviouristic data should be collected primarily for the purpose of analysing the functions of mental life. *Every momentary mental state should then be interpreted as an unfinished act with the overt completion of the act as a basis of interpretation.*

5. A Motivistic Interpretation of Mind

In Fig. 4 I have represented in schematic form an interpretation of mental life as unfinished action. The sequence from the sources of the dynamic living self to its expression in conduct is represented by the vertical down-ward direction of the diagram. Time is represented by the dimension from left to right. Let us assume that the natural state of living is activity, the expression of the life-energy of the organism into action, random or purposive action, useful or useless action. The fundamental problem of psychology is to study this sequence from as near to the source as we can explore to the seen conduct by which we live and by which we are judged. Since we know very little about the sources or mainsprings of conduct we must necessarily be vague about their exact nature. We may call them instincts or motives or impulses to live. In the diagram I have labelled them as instincts.

The impulse is not subject to conscious control or even conscious recognition in its entire course toward expression. It is only in the latter part of the expression of an impulse that it is subject to conscious participation. The first phase of the impulse is probably what we know as the subconscious. According to this interpretation the subconscious is in a sense preconscious or precognitive in that the impulse has not taken on sufficient definiteness to become conscious content. At this stage the impulse has as its sole attributes affective characteristics which are too diffuse and unlocalized to be even introspectively identified. The course of the impulse through this early phase of its expression is not subject to the control of willed guidance and choice ; it is not conscious in any focal sense, and it cannot be controlled by rational judgment. It is only when the impulse has defined itself considerably into the form of an idea, a concept, a proposed general line of conduct, that it is subject to further definition by means of rational guidance. Rational control is, however, limited even here to the acceptance and rejection of the ideas that occur to us. Ideas are never produced and formed by rational control.

As the impulse emerges from the preconscious phase of its

history with a minimum of attributes, it constitutes a concept or higher thought process. It is higher in the sense that it is loosely organized, vague, incomplete with reference to the action that it may lead to. It contains very little to identify it. It points only to a type of action to which it may lead. It is in this sense that we can say that the higher thought processes are closer to the subconscious or preconscious than the perceptual processes. Of course it is not necessary for an impulse to emerge from the subconscious phase of its history at the conceptual stage. It may not emerge in focal consciousness until it has been almost completely formed into a percept, an act that is almost ready to be completed. *What we know as consciousness is the presence of impulses that have been more or less defined and which conflict with each other, and thus arrest their own expression.* The conflicts of impulses that are rather well specified constitute consciousness in a functional sense. Impulses clash no doubt in their earlier, less particularized phase when they are little more than affective trends, when they have not been defined sufficiently to be the subject of conscious inspection and reflection. Such conflicts give rise to feeling states of a temporary or a permanent kind which in aggravated forms constitute the mystery of the neuroses.

An act which is entirely automatic is the expression of an impulse which in its course of particularization meets no conflicting impulse and therefore does not become conscious. It issues straight into action. An instinctive act is the expression of an impulse, usually strong, which does not meet with any interference until it reaches the perceptual stage of completion. It differs from a reflex mainly in that conscious participation in the instinctive act appears at the perceptual stage of completion. It is less predictable as to its final details than the reflex. It is subject to conscious and rational guidance at its perceptual stage of formation. An impulse which is arrested by conflicts while it is still loosely formed constitutes imagery and thinking in a higher sense. *Higher and lower forms of mental life differ, then, mainly in that the higher mental processes involve the conflict of impulses that are as yet only loosely formed, whereas simpler or lower forms of mental life consist in the conflicts of impulses that are fairly well specified.* In the animal mind we have the capacity for conflict of impulses and conscious guidance at the perceptual stage when the impulses contain the perceptual specifications of the immediate present. Mental power and intelligence consist in the capacity for allowing the rough, vague, loose, almost intangible impulses to clash before they have become particularized into percepts or definitely specified ideas. In the diagram this would be represented by continuing the parallel lines of the conscious stream farther up toward the sources of activity. But not even the genius can push his control of ideas, of partially formulated impulses, clear up to the source. He must wait for them to appear already partly specified. That phase of formulation through which the idea passes before it emerges for conscious verification and evaluation is the subconscious or preconscious. That moment of transition when the impulse or idea is confidently known to be there but at which we cannot see it, know it, or say it—when it is only experienced as feeling, but not yet within our control, that moment marks the stage at which the impulse or idea is taking on sufficient attributes to become cognitively known. We have no guarantee that the idea, when it does appear, will be a cognitive universal, a concept. It may appear with a rush, well formulated into the imaginal or perceptual stage of completion. In that case it may be recognized as a clever idea, but it will not be a higher thought process unless it appears with only just enough attributes to constitute a line of conduct, a universal which needs much further particularization before it can issue into conduct.

My main idea is that mental life can be thought of as action in the process of being formulated. Any particular mental state can be thought of as an act that is unfinished, an impulse which in its course of particularization is in conflict with some other impulse. The higher thought processes would be impulses toward action that are as yet only loosely defined with a minimum of intension and a maximum of extension. The several cognitive categories can be interpreted as differing mainly and in a functional sense in the degree of completion of the act. Higher and abstract mental life is loosely organized and anticipates a *type* of conduct rather than the specific act. The definition attained by an impulse or motive before it becomes conscious constitutes the subconscious or preconscious. If this interpretation is correct, the subconscious is continuous with consciousness, an impulse being preconscious before it becomes conscious. Mental life would be interpreted in the light of the action into which it completes itself. It would not merely represent action. Mental life would actually *be* action in unfinished form.

6. Consciousness as a Particularizing Function

In the previous sections I have insisted that every mental state is unfinished action. Mental life must of course become finished action if it is to be biologically justifiable. I shall postulate a universal tendency of every mental state to particularize itself. By this I mean that every psychological object tends automatically to take on additional attributes, to specify itself more concretely, and thereby to become motorially more complete. *To think is to add new attributes to that which we are thinking about.* This means an increase of intension and a decrease of extension of the psychological object. This also means that the psychological object naturally and without conscious effort tends to specify itself toward the motorium.

Stop now and notice what really constitutes your concept "house". If you dwell on that concept you will discover that, unless you specially guard against it, you will be imagining a particular house; you are perhaps directly in front of it, or you are in it right now. You even " see " the furniture and rugs—in this that was a concept when you started. I grant that this particularized imagery may *serve* as a concept, as a carrier of the fewer attributes that characterize the universal. But the fact remains that this minutely specified imagery is not itself a concept. The concept is a very unstable entity, and it is biologically well that it should be. The concept is a sign with a few hints on it, and it points in some other direction than the one in which we are looking. If its few attributes fit the purpose of the moment, we look farther in its direction so as to see more of its attributes—until we see all of them. When we do that we foresee where that concept leads to, and we express it in action by following, by rejecting, by continuing in the line of least resistance, or by waiting for another sign to appear.

The concept " house " does not normally appear unless we have some want which tends to become satisfied by an adjustment concerning a house. In Fig. 4 the concept would be represented by one of the upper parallel lines which are labelled "higher thought processes". The impulse is in its early and incomplete stage of expression. The undulating line which is marked " particularization " represents the course of an impulse toward final expression in adjustment. At several stages, the impulse becomes conscious successively in conceptual terms, in ideational terms, and in perceptual terms. The expression of the impulse is in one sense an accretion of attributes. The higher cognitive forms of the impulse are incompletely specified, while its lower cognitive forms are more definitely specified. Progress toward the right on the chart means time and delay in neutralizing the impulse. Progress downward on the chart means the universal ideo-motor tendency.

Let us consider the particularizing effect in perception. You have a club sandwich before you. The percept of that sandwich is the unfinished act of eating it, or otherwise disposing of it. The percept tends to take on new attributes if it is mentally at all sustained. The first glance at the sandwich does not contain in it the attributes of eating with the fingers or with knife and fork. The percept, even when so defined, does not contain in it the attributes specifying which half of the sandwich is to be eaten first ; the normal function of perception is to add new attributes until the percept is so completely specified that it becomes an overt adjustment. In Fig. 4 we should represent the perceptual stages of the psychological act at the lower parallel lines which are close to the motorium.

Suppose that you have been aroused to a fit of violent temper against another man. Your behaviour would be said to be instinctive. Your motive is to injure him and if the instinctive pressure is strong your motive will be particularized to the perceptual stage without conscious guidance. The instinctive act of striking him has defined itself through the conceptual and ideational stages auto-matically. The motive appears in focal consciousness first when it has reached the perceptual stage. The instinctive act of striking is keenly conscious in that it is perceptually guided. This is represented diagrammatically by the line which is labelled " instinctive action ". Note that this motive does not become conscious at the early and higher cognitive stages. It becomes conscious first when it needs perceptual aid in order to be effective. The perceptual guidance of the striking act limits the act to one of immediate conscious purpose.

Let us return to the situation of being stuck on a country road with an engine that refuses to work. Up until this moment your motive in its more immediate sense was to go, and since it was being satisfied you lent only the slight perceptual guidance required to stay on the road and to move on. That motive is frustrated. The motive " to go " now becomes keenly conscious, and it tries to find satisfaction by defining itself in different tentative imaginal ways. It is at this stage that the stimulus appears. The stimuli such as the sound and appearance of the engine and the kinesthetic stimuli, all share in determining which of various concepts and ideas are to appear in the mind of the driver. Certain combinations of stimuli would cause the motive to express itself as the concept " ignition ". When this concept appears it is an incomplete act of starting to go again. The concept has no sooner appeared than it particularizes itself by adding such new attributes as " ignition plus spark plug ", and then appears, perhaps, " ignition plus spark plugs plus third cylinder plus dirty, etc." This process requires often only a fractional part of a second. The particularization continues until some inconsistency arises when it is no longer identified with our purposes.

The driver then waits for another idea to appear. Perhaps the next concept to appear is " gas supply ". This normally defines itself by additional attributes such as " gas supply plus empty tank plus so far to the next farmhouse plus walking plus looking to see if this is so ". The concept has defined itself to the perceptual stage. At this stage the motive in its ideational form drives one to look for the stimulus by which to complete the idea in action. Suppose that this line of thought is found inconsistent by the presence of gasolene in the tank. It is now possible to let the concept " gas supply " reappear in order to define itself along some other route, as, for example, " gas supply plus carburetor plus clogged carburetor." When the concept defines itself toward action it loses its characteristics as a concept by becoming particularized. In all of these cases the concepts appear as tentative outlets for the motive " to go again ".

Every mental state is biologically to be considered as unfinished action. The interpretation of our mental life is most profitably made on the basis of the adjustments which it mediates. We are already familiar with the generally accepted principle that mental states tend to express themselves in action sooner or later. But this principle has not been given the necessary emphasis. We are in the habit of accepting it as an interesting fact but not as a fundamental guide for the interpretation of conscious life. What I am proposing is, therefore, again only a shift of emphasis.

Another generally accepted principle in psychology is that of ideo-motor action. By this we usually understand the automatic and impulsive transition of an idea or percept into action. I should suggest the use of this term for the universal tendency of every mental state to define itself by additional attributes until it precipitates in action. What we ordinarily understand by ideo-motor action would then be a special case of a principle that is universal for all conscious life.

I should propose the term particularization to refer to the effect of the ideo-motor tendency on the psychological object. The ideo-motor tendency would then be the tendency of mental states to express themselves in action. Particularization would describe the changes in the psychological object, brought about by the ideo-motor tendency. *Of course the ideo-motor tendency does not in any sense explain itself. The term only brings to our attention the fact that the tendency is universal.*

CHAPTER IV

STAGES OF THE REFLEX CIRCUIT

1. THE ADJUSTMENT

When we are thinking and writing about the simplest kind of action, the reflex, we find it expedient to split it into the familiar temporal sequence of a stimulating cause and a reflex response. This agrees with a demonstrable material neurological relation. Since there is evident correspondence between the temporal sequence of events, as we see them, and the neurological machinery by which the reflex is carried, we extend the same language with some hypothetical additions to the more deliberate forms of conduct. In deliberate and intelligent conduct we assume that the neurological correlates become correspondingly more complex but that their general pattern remains essentially the same with reference to these three phases—the stimulating cause, a modifying mental set of the actor, and a terminal in the act as seen. When the act is quite complex, or when the concept of the reflex is applied to continuous adaptive conduct, we speak of the reflex circuit instead of the reflex arc to indicate the fact that the adjustment is itself, in a sense, the starting-point for continued adjustment.

Let us apply the idea of the reflex circuit to the mental history of an act. I have said elsewhere that we may dethrone the stimulus as a starting-point for conduct and promote the individual person himself to that responsibility, giving him the use of his environment as his perceptual tools with which to live. We may consider mental life as unfinished action, conduct in the process of being formulated. The total sequence of the development of an impulse originating in the person himself, defining itself through the perceptual present and issuing completed in the form of overt behaviour, may be thought of as a psychological act. The psychological act is to be distinguished from an act in the usual sense in that a seen act is the terminal of the psychological act, the end point in the development of an impulse, a present issue or completion which a moment before was unformed and mental. The reflex circuit would apply to the route by which the psychological act travels. Its description would tell us something of the typical stages and turning points at which mental life formulates itself into conduct.

The logical procedure would be to start at the beginning of the circuit and to describe the successive parts of the road, as it were, the successive typical stages by which an impulse becomes real action. But that would be to start with what is necessarily vague and unknown, action which is so unformed that it contains no introspectively distinguishable attributes at all. It is better, therefore, to start the description at the terminal end, the end of the circuit which is definitely known to common sense, and to trace its course backward as far as we can go.

By adjustment we mean simply seen behaviour and, possibly, glandular activity as well. There is nothing necessarily mental about the adjustment itself, but it becomes of psychological interest in that all mental life is adjustment in the process of being formed. The psychological categories which immediately precede overt behaviour are perception and sensation. In these categories we shall find the adjustment almost completed, but not sufficiently specified, to issue into conduct without some further delimitation. The central interest in the category of perception and sensation is to note the typical ways in which, at this stage of the psychological act, the impulse to activity becomes sufficiently delimited to become conduct as judged by the environment. The other cognitive categories, the so-called higher ones, concern the impulse to activity, the impulse to live, when it is even less definitely specified, when it does not contain enough attributes to constitute even a percept.

2. PERCEPTION AND THE STIMULUS

When a motive or impulse expresses itself into action without conscious participation we call the act an automatic one. It may be either the random expression of the activity which constitutes living at a moment when no particular purpose is urgent, or it may be the expression of a fully formed habit expressing itself without conscious or purposive guidance. The next step in increasing psychological complexity is the non-conscious particularization of an impulse until it reaches the perceptual stage of the psychological act. It then becomes subject to perceptual guidance which is conscious and rational between the limits of the perceptually given present. The general nature of the adjustment is at least partly specified, and that which constitutes the percept indicates in what ways the unformed action still remains to be defined.

Perception may be thought of as particularized sensation. *The percept is a motorially defined sense-impression.* The ideo-motor tendency from sensation to perception is so strong that it is exceedingly difficult to maintain a sense-quality without giving it the motorial interpretation which constitutes perception. If we consider the history of the psychological act, especially as regards its degree of completeness, we find that perception is action almost completely formed and that sensation is a still less specified, an earlier stage of the act. This is represented diagrammatically in Fig. 5.

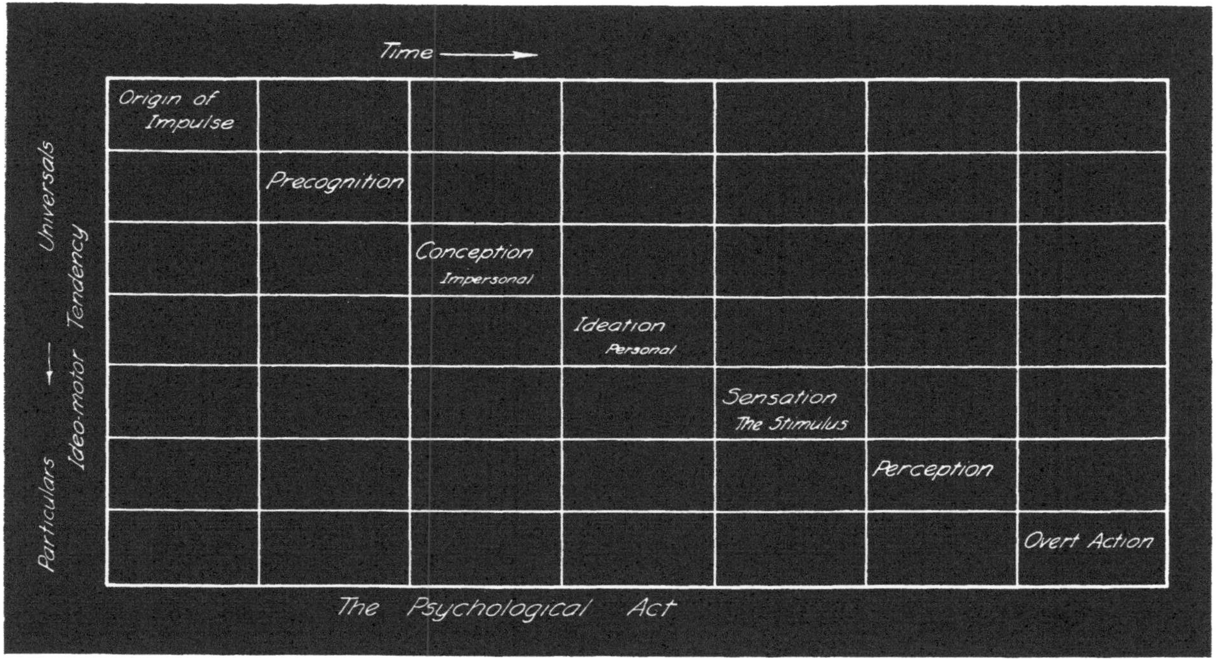

Fig. 5.

[To face p. 60.

3. IDEATION AND CONCEPTION

Where is the impulse or motive before the stimulus
is found ? It is either a readiness to act in a satisfying
way, or else it is focal in ideational form. One is a latent
state while the other is an active one. One refers to
a potential purpose while the other refers to a purpose
that is active. The purpose may or may not be conscious.
We are here using the term motive as more or less
synonymous with impulse. It may be conscious or
unconscious. We express our gregariousness, for example,
whenever there is perceptual provocation for it, and sometimes we seek the stimuli for expressing it. A man walks
into my office and says " Good Morning ", and I answer.
I was entirely willing to see him before he entered, but my
willingness was not necessarily focal. The perceptual
presence of the man simply gave suitable opportunity
to express my willingness in action. My willingness to
be agreeable was there before the stimulus.

The other form in which the motive may exist before
the stimulus appears is focal and ideational. When I am
working at my desk, it may occur to me that I should
like to see that man. This idea may express itself by
grasping the telephone or by going to his office. The
various stimuli are then either sought for or, if encountered
unexpectedly, they are perceived in terms of my present
purpose to see him. The idea is a motive or impulse in
its unfinished and pre-perceptual stage. *The idea is the
imaginal representation of an expected experience,* and
it contains fewer attributes than the corresponding

perceptual experience itself. The idea is a tentative course of action and is subject to trial-and-error inhibition or expression depending on its consistency with the momentary purpose. The idea may be considered as a turning point in the definition of the motive which allows greater latitude and better control of its expression than a perceptual form of the same motive. A motive may define itself automatically to the perceptual stage, or it may become focal earlier when it has fewer attributes and appears as an idea.

The concept is similar to the idea except that it contains fewer attributes. I find it profitable to draw a distinction between the concept and the idea in that the idea contains enough attributes to define one's bodily relation in the imaginally expected experience, whereas the concept does not. If my imaginal representation of " newspaper " contains enough attributes to specify whether I am imagining myself holding a newspaper, reading it, tearing it, looking at it, talking to a reporter, or otherwise imagining my bodily relation to the psychological object, the representation should be called an idea. If, on the other hand, my representation of " newspaper " is simply the visual or articulatory imagery of the word, a something which means publicity, or " bad ", or the carrier of public opinion, without containing enough attributes at the moment to specify my bodily relations to the psycho-logical object, then the imaginal representation should be spoken of as a concept. *The concept is a motive, caught and rendered focal so early in its expression that it does not yet contemplate our own bodily situation in the imaginally expected experience. The concept is an unfinished act so skeletal that our own bodily location still remains to be chosen.* In this sense the concept is impersonal while, in the same sense, the idea is personally defined. The latitude in choice of adjustment is considerably extended by the capacity to guide our motives before they are even personally defined. These various stages of the reflex circuit are represented diagrammatically in Fig. 5.

4. PRECOGNITION

It sometimes happens that we want something without being able to say just what it is that we want. We feel dissatisfied with our situation, but we are unable to state what it is that would satisfy us. This attitude of mind is discernible by unusual shifts in what we might call our interest limens or interest thresholds for different topics. We *feel* our motive without being able to make it focal. The only way in which the motive can be at all inferred in such a state of mind is to note the attitudes of appetition or aversion to different ideas, images, and topics of conversation. This is a stage in the expression of the motive that may be designated pre-cognitive. There is nothing in one's focal consciousness that definitely identifies the motive. And yet the motive makes its presence felt by favouring certain topics and discouraging others. The motive in this stage is, however, particularized to this extent that it favours a certain group of topics and inhibits other topics. This constitutes a kind of definition by elimination and that is what the subsequent particularizations in focal consciousness are also.

There is one sense in which the precognitive stage of the motive is indicative of at least momentary failure. The delimitations of the motive in its precognitive stage are not subject to mental trial-and-error choice. The specification of the want or need at this stage is subject to random definition. In this way a series of ideas occur until one appears which is consistent with the momentary purpose. Its further elaboration is subject to rational selection and control.

Suppose that a man is designing a machine part. He feels what he wants, but he is not able even to describe the nature of the design. He feels certain, however, that he could identify the design that he is looking for, if it were suggested to him. Usually these felt criteria are in the nature of operative conditions rather than descriptive of the machine detail. When the purpose is in this precognitive stage it is not yet sufficiently defined to be identified by any focal content even in conceptual terms. The same attitude may sometimes be found in a man who takes a position with administrative duties. He feels certain that something definite and desirable can be accomplished out of the mass of detail in which he is placed, but he would be unable to give a good account of himself if pressed at that time. He would be capable of expressing strong likes and dislikes about other comparable organizations depending on the similarity or dissimilarity to his own objective. But his own objective is not yet sufficiently defined to be completely specified in focal and cognitive terms. This objective is cognitive only in the sense that he has feelings of aversion and appetition toward groups or types of cognitive specifications. When this attitude is accompanied by strong feelings for or against large types of adjustment, it is probable that the felt objective will shortly become focal in more closely defined form although there is never any guarantee that this attitude will be fruitful. A distressing fact about this frame of mind is that it is not subject to rational solution. There is as yet nothing definitely focal to rationalize about. On the other hand, this attitude is not infrequently diagnostic of the appearance of a new solution.

If we are in the habit of applying the free-body principle to problems in mechanics, we define any such problem through this principle preconsciously so that the problem becomes focal with the attributes of this principle already attached. This makes for effective thinking because the application of the principle is then made without rational effort and choice.

If we have an exciting emotional experience, it is not unnatural that an attitude of aversion or avoidance should become habitual for some element in that experience. To find ourselves again in a similar situation is to experience fear and avoidance. The fear is part of the habitual perception of the situation. Since the fear is habitual the situation contains the fear when it becomes focal. Further rationalization can add new attributes but it cannot eradicate or reduce the attributes already in the motive when it became focal. To accomplish this, it is necessary to render the motive focal at an earlier, more abstract stage, before the fear-attribute has been added. If this can be done, rationalization along a non-fear route is possible. This is essentially what the psychoanalytic methods attempt to accomplish. They would make focal the fear-situation as it was before the fear was added. Let it then particularize itself along a non-fear solution and the mental habit is at least partially broken.

5. THE UNIVERSAL AND THE PARTICULAR IN THE PSYCHOLOGICAL ACT

The development of the reflex circuit can be spoken of as proceeding from the particular to the universal, and it can also be represented as proceeding from the universal to the particular. Since I have described the particularization of the circuit as an irreversible process in the direction from the universal to the particular, it may be advisable to make clear the manner in which the development of the circuit can also be represented as proceeding in the opposite direction. If we should describe the phylogenetic development of intelligence, we should begin by the perceptual intelligence of animals. Their mental life is primarily concerned with the particulars of perceptual experience. The intelligence of man is capable of imaginal anticipation of experience, and this anticipation is more universal than perceptual anticipation. The highest forms of intelligence involve conceptual thinking which is in terms of universals. This description traces a development from intelligence with particulars to intelligence which deals in universals and particulars. The same order would be appropriate for the genetic development of intelligence in man. The intelligence of children is first apparent in terms of particulars in perceptual experience. It develops later the capacity for imaginal representation of experience, and still later in more mature form with universals.

Whenever we are describing the genesis of intelligence we are tracing it from the particulars to the universals. But whenever we are concerned with the psychological act on any occasion, we must realize that the process is from universals to particulars. The perceptual intelligence of animals proceeds in the same direction when it is actually functioning. One of these considerations is with respect to the derivation and development of the intelligence, and the other consideration is with respect to the actual functioning of intelligence on any specific occasion. When the animal uses his intelligence in the form of distance-perception, he is making focal an adjustment in terms of the distance-impressions, particularizing them toward the overt act which is relatively more particular than the distance-impression with which he starts the conscious specification of the overt act. It is the same with human intelligence at work. If we get an idea by which to resolve a difficulty, this idea can be considered as a universal relative to the particularization of it toward the overt act. Whenever we are describing the intelligent act as such, we are describing an irreversible process which always proceeds from the universal to the particular. But when we are describing the genetic development of this capacity, we are describing the intelligent act as starting explicitly farther and farther back towards the universals.

In Fig. 6 I have represented this distinction. Even in

the lowest form of the intelligent act, as it may be seen in the mental life of animals, we have the motive particularizing itself toward the adjustment. This process is from universals to particulars even though the universal by which the adjustment becomes focal is of a relatively low order. In imaginal intelligence we have the same irreversible process from universals to particulars, with this difference that the process becomes focal earlier in the act. This genetic development is represented graphically by moving the focus to the left in the diagram. This means that the starting-point for the conscious particularization of the act is moved toward universals of higher order.

Finally we have conceptual intelligence, which, when it is in operation, functions irreversibly from the universals to the particulars just as in animal intelligence. The difference is primarily that the focal point in the particularizing process has moved to universals of still higher order. It should be clear, then, that intelligence at work always proceeds from universals to particulars, but that the genetic development of intelligence marks a progress in moving the focal point from particulars, or universals of low order, toward universals of higher order.

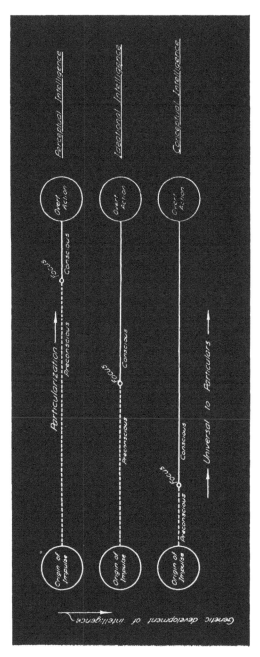

F<small>IG</small>. 6.

[*To face p. 68.*

CHAPTER V

THE PRINCIPLE OF PROTECTIVE ADJUSTMENT

1. THE RECEPTORS AND BODILY RISK

The phylogenetic development of intelligence can be unified in what we may call the principle of protective adjustment. The application of intelligence in any form of adjustment is an effort to satisfy the wants of the organism with the least possible physical risk. This applies not only to the higher forms of intelligent conduct in man but it applies as well to animal intelligence.

An organism which has no differentiated sense-organs is compelled to expose its main body to the unknown conditions of the environment in satisfying its wants. Such an organism is not able to explore the environment except by coming in bodily contact with the environmental facts. This limitation is made still more serious if the organism possesses no differentiated contact receptors which can be sent out to explore the unknown situation before exposing the main body to it. It should be obvious that such an organism satisfies the wants of its normal life at considerable risk to its physical self.

Consider the advantage of the organism which is equipped with exploring members such as vibrissæ or tentacles. These protect the main body trunk and can be used to explore an environmental situation before exposing the main body to it. Such differentiated receptors constitute landmarks in the phylogenetic development of intelligence. The development of sense-organs is continuous with the very highest forms of human intelligence. The sense-impressions from the exploring member have biological value only in so far as they are identified by the animal with the equivalent contact experience which would be encountered if the sense-impressions were ignored. To perceive, then, by means of an exploring member is to equate the sense-impression with the equivalent contact experience. If that expected contact experience fits with the momentary purpose, the adjustment issues into overt form. If the sense-impressions disagree with the momentary purpose the sense-impressions are either ignored or avoided by turning in some other direction for different stimuli. Even the lowest forms of differentiated contact receptors give the animal some control over future time and over distance. In these respects the efficiency afforded by the contact receptors is of the same variable as the efficiency which we claim by our human intelligence or foresight. The contact receptors have their biological justification in the increased facility for satisfying bodily wants with a minimum of bodily exposure and risk.

It is of course obvious that the distance receptors serve the same purpose as the contact receptors except that the control is extended still more into future time and distance.

In this sense there is a psychological identity between future time and space. Smell is a distance-sense department which has its nearest correlate in the contact-sense department of taste. To perceive by smell is to live imaginally the expected taste experience. The smell percept is in fact the imaginal equivalent of the contact experience of taste. The contact experience is accordingly consummated, ignored, or avoided, depending on the momentary purposes.

This equivalence of the sense-impressions through the distance and contact receptors is obvious enough as far as smell and taste are concerned. The equivalence for vision or hearing and their corresponding contact experiences is not so often noted.

Consider at random any visual percept such as the percept of a knife. To perceive the knife is to feel ready to pick it up, to handle it, to use it. If the surface of the blade looks smooth, this visual smoothness and polish are perceived as expected smoothness to the touch and expected ease of cutting. To perceive through the distance receptors is to live imaginally the expected contact experience.

The term " meaning " covers the particularization of the sense-impression that I am here discussing. It is, however, not adequate to consider meaning as though it were simply an equation or symbolic representation. The meaning of the visual impressions from the knife is not simply a lot of details that are equated to the visual impression. It is not adequate to say that the sense-impression A " means " B, C, D, in the form of an equation. The sense-impression A *completes* itself by *adding* attributes which become an imaginal contact experience. It should be clear that meaning does not refer merely to associated attributes. It refers to the ever-present ideo-motor tendency of sense-impressions to particularize themselves into expected experience. If these imaginal experiences fit our momentary purposes we live them out into overt form. If they do not fit our various motives at the moment we ignore or inhibit the execution of the meaning. If we interpret the term "meaning" in this way we bring it into line with a mind that works, and not merely with an abstract description of associated mental elements. The term "meaning" is in a sense synonymous with particularization with the exception that in its ordinary use it is restricted to a narrower range of definition of the psychological object than what I have tried to convey by the term "particularization".

I should like to call attention to the fact that Vierordt's law with reference to local sign can be related to the principle of protective adjustment. Vierordt's law states that the local sign discrimination is keenest in those skin surfaces which are farthest removed from the joints and body trunk and which are most movable. The biological justification for this type of discrimination is probably in the increased facility for exploring the environment. It is therefore consistent that we should find this type of discrimination keenest on the skin surfaces of the exploring members of the body. It is keener on the finger tips than on the forearm, keener there than on the shoulder, and keener there than on the back.

Consider yourself walking in the dark. You would perhaps use the foot as an exploring member before trusting your body weight on it. This protects the main body from the unknown conditions into which you would step. If you have a cane handy it would be used as an exploring member by which the unknown conditions of the immediate future could be controlled with the least possible bodily risk. If a flash-light were available, it would give more facility in controlling the immediate future, and it would enable you to inhibit false steps without ever executing them. With daylight the expected contact experience can be roughly anticipated even hours before it is encountered. That is what visual perception actually consists of, namely the partial living through of the consummatory act with its consequences.

2. RECEPTORS AND THE CONTROL OF FUTURES

The contact and distance receptors show an increase of control over the environment in the expression of bodily wants. The next higher form in the development of intelligence is the capacity to imagine the desired stimulus before it is perceptually present even to the distance receptors. Suppose that you are driving along a country road and that you notice that your gasolene supply is getting low. The thought may become focal in a fleeting way that you will stop at the next gasolene station. When the next gasolene station becomes visible you may be thinking and talking about entirely different things, but since the motive to get some more gasolene has not yet been satisfied you are more than ordinarily sensitive to stimuli with such reference. The sign as a stimulus therefore becomes focal. Shortly after you have filled the gasolene tank you may pass other stations without even seeing the signs. Your sensitivity for that kind of stimulus is then low because there is not in you any unsatisfied motive which can express itself through the subsequent signs.

Suppose that you have on several occasions been vaguely dissatisfied with the disorderly appearance of your current magazines and catalogues which you now have in a heap on top of a table. They do not present the orderly appearance which would be consistent with that of your other belongings. You may never have stopped to consider any remedy. You may never even have made any comment about it. You are walking along the sidewalk with a friend discussing the events of the day. Your office is not focal and perhaps not even marginal. Nevertheless you stop at an office furniture window to look at a filing case which might be suitable for the orderly keeping of the magazines and catalogues. In this case an unsatisfied motive, the expression or solution of which has never been focal, constitutes the source of an unusual sensitivity to those stimuli which might serve to particularize and express that motive. You may never have thought of a special filing case for your magazines and catalogues, and yet your feeling of dissatisfaction about their appearance would make you sensitive to those stimuli which might constitute suitable particularizations of the motive or dissatisfaction.

These two illustrations show that the motive, which is simply an unsatisfied want, is primarily responsible for our sensitiveness to the stimuli of the environment. The motive may have been focal as an expressed want. This was the case in the gasolene illustration. The motive may have been focal simply as a dissatisfaction with reference to some psychological object without being developed far enough to make focal any proposed expression or solution of it. That was the case with the dissatisfaction about the magazines. There is no sharp line of demarcation between these. They differ only in the extent to which the motive has been particularized when it was last focal. *It is essential to keep in mind that the motive and the percept are not two different things. The percept is simply the more completely defined motive.* The appearance of the stimulus can be interpreted as synonymous with the attitude, " Look, this is the particular way in which I might satisfy my want." The perceptual presence of the stimulus is a partial delimitation and expression of the motive. The interest or attention that we give to a stimulus depends first of all on its possibility as an avenue of expression for our desires.

Most of the stimuli that we encounter in our everyday life are actually looked for. The motive defines itself along some avenue and becomes focal as a psychological object which is then searched for by more or less random or guided moving about. When the stimulus is found, it consists of the searched-for psychological object and the perceptual detail around it serves further to define the overt expression of the motive. For example, you are about to leave your house and it is the time of the first cold weather of the winter. You decide to use your fur cap. Your motive has become particularized as the verbal imagery of the fur cap and you search for that stimulus. On your way to the wardrobe you expect to find the stairway, which serves as a stimulus to step on it ; you expect to find the switch in the wardrobe which serves as stimulus to turn on the light. Most of the stimuli that we encounter are expected either focally or marginally.

The capacity to expect a stimulus before it is present obviously has survival value. We are fortunate in this capacity because we can satisfy our wants not only in terms of the piece of environment with which we are actually now in contact, and through the neighbouring environment which we partly control through our distance receptors, but also through the imaginally expected stimuli into which our purposes have defined themselves and which we can set about systematically to look for.

Ideation is the process of putting detail into our motives. Ideation is in this respect the process of completing that which starts at the motive end of the reflex circuit. There is another aspect of ideation with reference to the terminal end of the circuit to which I should like also to call attention. Ideation is not only to be considered as the process of completing or defining the motive. Every idea has a retrospective reference to its source in a motive or dissatisfaction, and it has also a forward or anticipatory reference to that which we expect to experience. Ideation is in this sense as close as possible a statement of that which we should like to experience, or that which we expect to face.

There is not infrequently in the mind of the student of psychology a misunderstanding regarding the difference between perception and imagination. It is often thought that perception is solely the sense-impressions with the attributes to which they are equated, and that imagination is something different in that it does not start with or depend on a perceptually present provocation. One is supposed to be externally caused, and the other is supposed to be internally caused. This is a cleavage between these two psychological categories which does not in reality exist. The misunderstanding is probably caused by the misinterpretation of what is to be included in the category of " meaning ". Practically all of the function of perception is imaginal. It is imaginal, to be sure, on a very completely defined stage. Perception may be treated as a form of imagination which is primarily kinesthetic in its reference and close to the motorium. The only part of the perception which is not imaginal is the sense-impression, but if the perceiving is at all intelligent the sense-impression elaborates readily into an imaginal contact experience with the perceived object. *The essential part of the percept is the imaginal experience with the perceived object.* The sense-impression is merely a cue defining the final detail of the contemplated act.

Consider the visual sense-impression from the sign " This way out " with an arrow-head indicating the direction. The sense-impression is here only a cue which helps to particularize the final muscular detail of my purpose to get out. The kinesthetic and visual imagery of completing this purpose is the essential part of the percept. The sense-impressions from the sign are only a relatively trivial part of the perceiving. The course of the imaginal anticipation of completing the purpose to get out is delimited by the sense-impression. It is a short cut by which one avoids both mental and overt trial and error. The sensorial cue serves as one of the final delimiting agents in the definition of the purpose.

It is of course possible to perceive without expecting either imaginally or by intention to complete any overt adjustment involving the perceived object. For example, you may perceive a small dot on a sheet of paper without having any intention to do anything about it. You may insist that you are perceiving in this case without entertaining any imaginal contact experience with the paper and the dot. You are correct. If you persist in perceiving the dot you will do so by adding attributes to the sensorial cue which were not present at its first appearance. You will think, perhaps, like this : " dot, round dot, pencil dot, it is so far away, it is in the middle of the sheet of paper, I see it clearly now, the light reflects on one side of the dot, I wonder if it punched through the paper," and so on. These additional attributes all look aimlessly toward completion of some sort. All this aimless perceiving is admittedly possible, but if in our daily life we should indulge in very much of this psychological laboratory perception, we should not long be allowed to take care of ourselves.

It is entirely possible for us to exercise our mental machinery on exhibit, as it were, without having any purpose in mind. One can do the same thing with a machine. You may punch the keys and levers of an adding machine just to show that you *can* operate the machine without having any need for it just now. That does not disprove that the machine has a normal purpose for which it was built. It is just so with mental life. We may sit in a psychological laboratory and prove by universal consensus that we can have mental operations without any purpose or objective whatever. That does not prove that our normal images, ideas, and thoughts, are not expressions of our purposes and wants. It is even possible to look at the dot and to inhibit the natural ideo-motor tendency of the sense-impression to particularize itself by adding new attributes. That is called auto-hypnosis and the result is that focal consciousness disappears altogether.

The fundamental difference between imagination and perception is that imagination precedes perception in the reflex circuit. Let us limit ourselves for the moment to imagination of the ideational sort in which concretely specified situations are imagined. Perception is closer to the motorium, and imagination is closer to the universal end of the definition of the motive. The *development of intelligence is measurable by the incompleteness of the motive at which it can become focal.* If the motive becomes focal as an imaginal experience before the stimulus has even appeared, the animal has in consequence of this capacity an increased control in the satisfaction of its wants with minimum risk. To imagine is to anticipate mentally the detailed experience by which the motive would be neutralized. Such a state of mind lowers the threshold for relevant stimuli and these can then be searched for with greater flexibility of adjustment than if the animal were compelled to wander about at random in the hope of stumbling over a promising stimulus. *Imagination can be thought of as the capacity to define a motive to the stage of a concrete experience by which the motive would be satisfied, and the capacity to do this without the assistance of the stimulus.* In a less mature form of intelligence the motive would express itself to the point of vague dissatisfaction issuing into random overt

running about. This level of intelligence would be capable
of particularizing the motive in terms of the present stimulus
when found, but it would not be capable of particularizing
the motive to the point of a concrete experience in the
absence of the stimulus. The process is essentially the same
in kind. The difference is only in the degree of incompleteness of the motive at which it becomes focal, and the capacity
to particularize the motive without the assistance of the
perceptually present particulars. *Imagination is identical
with perception with the sensorial cue omitted.* The mind that
we are here discussing is progressing to higher and higher
intelligence in that the motive becomes focal at earlier and
earlier stages in the circuit when it contains fewer and fewer
attributes. At the highest levels of intelligence we shall
have the motive becoming focal when it contains only those
attributes which define it as a universal.

3. ABSTRACTION AS CONTROL OF FUTURES

Let us consider conceptual thinking as a form of protective
adjustment. You are going to send a parcel to someone in
another city. Will you send it express, or by the ordinary
mail, or by parcel post ? When you think of your purpose
" to send the package " you are in reality entertaining a
purpose which is still unformed. If there is absolutely no
conflict of impulses regarding the details of the act of
sending the parcel you will not even stop to think about it.
But as the specific acts by which you are about to send the
package are just about to be completed, the unformed
action is mental in its conceptual terms. The incomplete

act " to send the package " defines itself successively in the three ways of sending it, and these are themselves concepts of lower order in that they are more defined, they contain more attributes than the arrested action at which they started. To think, even in so simple a situation as this, means to strip the final action as far as possible of the details which are not absolutely essential to identify it, and to be ready to repeat the process if the fortuitous particularization is not entirely satisfactory. Let us suppose that you decide to send the package by express. The decision to do so involves the partial definition of a concept which is still a concept of a lower order. Even at that moment your mental state does not perhaps contain in it the elements to determine whether the package is to be sent now or to-morrow morning, whether you will take it to the express office or telephone, and so on. As the action takes on sufficient details to involve your own bodily situation with reference to the expected experience, the mental state becomes an idea in the sense in which we have here defined it. The stimuli from the environment such as the sight of the telephone, the office, the appropriate label for the chosen manner of sending the package, these stimuli are expected and when found they help further to define the expected experience into reality.

Finally, let us consider the relationship between what has been called the recession of the stimulus and the principle of protective adjustment. The recession of the stimulus refers to the fact that with the advance of intelligence through the distance receptors and the capacity to imagine, we note effective adjustments being made in terms of more and more inconspicuous stimuli. The lowest animal forms must be in physical contact with their food before random search can be abandoned in favour of the guided precurrent or consummatory adjustments. The presence of smell organs enables the organism to abandon random search sooner, and to instal guided precurrent adjustments earlier in its search for the stimulus. The distance receptors of vision and hearing allow random search to be abandoned still earlier in favour of precurrent adjustments which are guided by the foresight of the distance receptors. This progress involves a diminution in the size of the sense-impression with reference to the receptor surface, and a decrease in the physical intensity of the stimulus itself. The same progress can also be thought of as a withdrawal of the animal body from the stimulus in time and space, allowing more and more opportunity for protective pre-current adjustment. This is synonymous with a reduction in the element of chance in the discovery of the stimulus. With the higher development of perceptual intelligence, and with rudimentary imaginative control, we have still more inconspicuous stimuli regarded by the animal as significant for guided precurrent adjustment. This is because the relatively insignificant features of the en vironment come to have what we know as meaning These insignificant features define themselves into expected experience. We credit intelligence as keen when we find it capable of inferring the rest of a situation from the trivial perceptual marks of it. It is not a far step to eliminate the insignificant stimulus altogether in defining our purposes to the point of imaginal concrete experience. *The recession of the stimulus is but another way of stating that increased intelligence means the increased capacity to express our wants with more and more independence of conspicuous and adjacent stimuli.*

In these illustrations I have shown that the development of intelligence can be thought of as continuous, beginning in the differentiation of structure of lower animal forms by which a portion of the body is set aside for the risky job of exploring the environment, protecting the body as far as possible. The development which is marked at first by material and objective mechanical differentiation of function leads in the mental development to the highest forms of intelligence in man, and it can be thought of as continuous in this sense that it is all concerned with the control of distance and its psychological equivalent, future time. The differentiated contact receptors serve as an immediate form of protection. The distance receptors extend considerably the same type of protection in that they enable the organism to ward off useless action before it even becomes incipient. As long as the animal is limited to contact receptors, the accepted as well as the rejected action must be more or less imminent or incipient before its value can be judged. With the aid of distance receptors the control is considerably extended into future time and space.

The major portion of perceptual activity is imaginal in that the expected experience for which the distance-impression serves as a cue is only very remotely contained in the distance-impression itself. Perception is largely imaginal in its nature. The distance-impression itself on the receptor surface is only a very slight and relatively insignificant portion of the experience of perceiving, compared with the imaginal or interpretative parts of it. It is therefore not a far step, after all, to realize that perceiving activity might well go on in its imaginal parts in the absence of the slight receptor stimulation. In this case we have imagination which is psychologically almost identical with perception except that it is less defined, less distinct, and more flexible to momentary alteration.

Let us now imagine the unfinished action which constitutes first perception, then, when still less defined, imagination, becoming less and less defined so that choices are made while the conflicting lines of conduct are still in their rough, general, loose, skeletal form, and we have conceptual thinking. *The less there is of the impulse at the time when it is subject to rational acceptance or rejection, the higher is the mentality of the actor.* Genius is essentially the capacity to deal effectively with impulses at the stage of formation when they are still only roughly defined affective states, before they have absorbed enough attributes to become the cognitive terms with which most of us are limited in our field of rational control. By the principle of protective adjustment I mean this unifying idea under which we can cover consistently the development of intelligence from its lowest forms to its highest, the development which gains for the organism increasing range of control of future action and consequently increasing security for the bodily self, a development which renders possible the choices of conduct which will find their overt execution in a more and more distant and removed future.

CHAPTER VI

THE PRECONSCIOUS PHASE OF THE REFLEX CIRCUIT

1. THE PRECONSCIOUS IMPULSE

I shall now describe the reflex circuit with special reference to what happens to the motive before it becomes completely conscious and focal. The motive passes through a process of particularization or specification in its development toward overt expression. By this I mean that the motive or impulse takes on new attributes until it becomes sufficiently specified to register as the immediately present adjustment. Before considering what we might call the pre-focal elaboration of the motive let us consider the progress that is usually made when some undertaking is planned and started with an original objective which is stated only as a universal.

Suppose that we are generally dissatisfied with the large number of accidents in some industrial establishment. There is need for something to be done but nothing has as yet been proposed. We are dissatisfied and perhaps worried about things as they are, but no effective adjustment has as yet been proposed even in imaginal form. Let us suppose that a committee is formed for the purpose of seeing if something can be done about it. Particular accidents are investigated to ascertain how they came about. The first constructive suggestion on the part of one of the members of the committee may be perhaps to erect signs at those points where the accidents seem to be particularly prevalent. When this idea occurs the dissatisfaction has become focal in the form of an idea which is to be imaginally lived through in order to ascertain whether it is consistent with the motive to reduce the frequency of accidents. One of the members of the committee may imagine a foreigner in the plant walking right into the dangerous situation because of his inability to read English. When that idea occurs it is an imaginal particularization of the idea to have danger signs, and this imaginal experience is an anticipated failure. The failure might by overt trial and error have been discovered, but in this case the failure of the idea to have danger signs is anticipated by living it through in anticipated imaginal experience. The dissatisfaction may be thought of as a pressure of social obligation and duty which becomes focal again in a slightly different form in the suggestion to have conspicuous red disks erected at the dangerous points throughout the plant. These signs would be intelligible to anyone irrespective of native language. This idea is lived

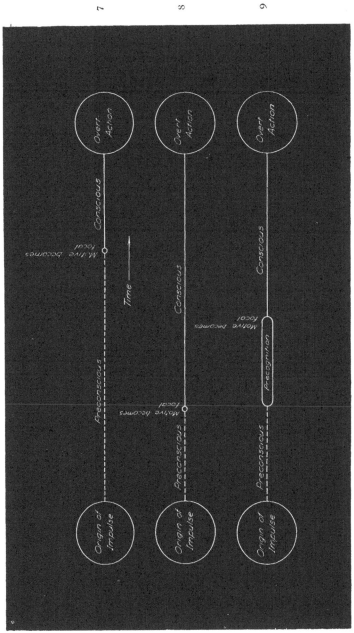

FIGS. 7, 8, AND 9.

[To face p. 86.

through by imagining how the place would look with these signs in appropriate places. If this imaginal particularization of the suggestion does not seem inconsistent it may be carried to completion in an overt adjustment, which would be the erection of the red disks.

Analyse this with reference to Fig. 7. I have indicated the motive or dissatisfaction at the extreme left of the diagram. This dissatisfaction is the driving force or motive power for the mental activities that are to express themselves in some suitable adjustment. There follows a time when the dissatisfaction is merely felt in terms of the cognitive evidence of the accidents. The first deliberations of the committee may consist merely in making clear what the dissatisfaction or need really is. The psychological interpretation of those deliberations would be that the dissatisfaction or problem is then being stated. To state a need in an intelligent manner is to strip from it the irrelevant details which may be inadvertently mixed with the dissatisfaction and which tend to obstruct an effective solution. If one of the members takes considerable time in the meetings of the committee to criticize the management in strong emotional terms, it would indicate that the need has perhaps not yet been closely defined unless his criticism is taken in the form of an analysis of the need itself. If another member recites the horrors of a particular accident without analysing its cause, he may be doing good service in stirring to action the feeling of social obligation on the part of other indifferent members of the committee. But such discussion may also have the detrimental effect of centering attention on the cognitive particulars about which the dissatisfaction is felt without aiding in the resolution of the problem and the task of the committee.

With reference to the solution of the problem or the attainment of the effective adjustment, this stage of the deliberations may be thought of as preceding the focal statement of an adjustment. The moment when the first constructive suggestion appears we have the resolution of the difficulty becoming focal. This constructive suggestion may be stated in the form of an idea which would be a concrete specification of the proposed adjustment. That would be the case if the suggestion were to erect a red sign at a particularly dangerous spot. The constructive suggestion by which the resolution becomes focal may appear on the other hand in conceptual form. That would be the case if the suggestion were to inaugurate some kind of instruction around the slogan " safety first ". That suggestion might not contain at its inception any details as to whether the instruction would be by pamphlets distributed in the pay envelope, or by lectures in different languages, or by moving pictures. None of these particulars may even have been thought of by the person who proposes a line of solution by education. Nevertheless, his suggestion would delimit to some extent the manner in which one might resolve the difficulty. The discussions preceding that suggestion might have been in the nature of a complete consideration of the difficulty in its various aspects, and a stripping of the problem of distracting particulars. The discussion which follows the constructive suggestion may be thought of as tentative adjustments stated in imaginal form and subject to mental trial-and-error choice.

Let us suppose that the final adjustment which is actually to be carried out is the exhibition of a series of moving pictures to show how easily an unsuspecting person may become the victim of a serious accident. Let us also suppose that the suggestion in the committee appears first as a proposal to educate the workmen in the precautions that they themselves might take. With reference to the adjustment which is actually to be carried out we may consider as preconscious all the deliberations that preceded the effective suggestion. The deliberations which follow the presentation of the suggestion may be thought of as conscious particularizations of the idea of education. These conscious particularizations are in reality the imaginal living through of the education idea in various forms in order that the most effective detailed educational adjustment may be selected.

2. IDEATIONAL AND CONCEPTUAL RESOLUTION OF THE IMPULSE

I have represented in Fig. 7 these stages in the reflex circuit and the point at which the motive or dissatisfaction becomes focal. By this I mean that the dissatisfaction is then stated in some imaginal form which is to be defined more closely by conscious delimitation. One may possibly object to this form of analysis by the statement that the preconscious stages of the motive are in reality conscious and are filled with cognitive terms which are perhaps even intensely focal. All that is granted. But *with reference to the effective adjustment* the deliberations preceding its focal statement are preconscious. They are the imaginal reinstatement perhaps of the dissatisfaction in all its various forms. They are in the nature of the expression, " Yes, all this is awful, we must do something about it. Jones was hurt yesterday—and then follows more detail—it is indeed an awful condition—what can we do about it ?—the management is indifferent—the men are careless— the foremen do not care—etc." All these discussions have their own focal content, to be sure, but with reference to the solution of this particular difficulty they precede the focal statement of the first proposed resolution of the trouble.

Briefly stated, Fig. 7 represents several stages in the cycle. First we have a felt need. Then we deliberate about the trouble or dissatisfaction. This is preliminary to the stage at which the first constructive suggestion appears. I call this stage of the psychological act preconscious with reference, of course, to the particular act by which this difficulty is to be resolved. The point at which the constructive suggestion appears is the moment at which the motive becomes focal. The motive is then no longer only a felt need. When it becomes focal it is more closely defined, and it then looks toward a type of adjustment by which the motive may be satisfied. The suggestion is the psychological act, arrived at the point of focal statement. From then on, we have the possibility of conscious control in that we can live the suggestion imaginally to its completion. If the concrete experience, so imaginally anticipated, promises to neutralize the dissatisfaction, it is acted out in overt form. If it does not seem to promise the disappearance of the dissatisfaction, it is dropped for lack of motive power. *We have then to consider in the analysis of the psychological act two main phases of it. We have first that irritation and discontent of a dissatisfied motive which gives by more or less random behaviour objective evidence of its presence. We have a second phase in which the motive has become focal and is attempting to express itself with sufficient delimitation to render possible the guidance of conscious elimination and choice. The point in the psychological act which separates those two main phases is the moment at which the motive becomes focal with reference to a proposed particular adjustment.*

In Figs. 7 and 8 I have shown the difference between the resolution of a problem when the imaginal tentative adjustment appears in the form of a universal, and when it appears as a particularized suggestion. In the previous illustrations I described the two possible types of suggestion by using as examples the proposal to erect a conspicuous red sign at a particular place, and the suggestion to start some programme of education to show the advantages of being careful. The former is a particularized suggestion whereas the latter is stated more in the form of a universal. In the diagrams I have shown the more particularized suggestion in Fig 7, and I have represented the suggested universal in Fig. 8, where the problem becomes focal at an earlier stage in the psychological act. It should be clear that if the psychological act becomes focal at an early stage, when the resolution is still very loosely defined, when the resolution is still in the form of a universal, the actor has a wide range of final adjustments among which to choose the particular expression of his desire. This makes for effectiveness in adjustment. By this capacity the actor has at his command many possible adjustments which do not even occur to the man whose suggestion is a particularized concrete experience imaginally represented. We may state as a principle with reference to intelligent conduct that *the earlier in the psychological act the motive becomes focal, the wider will be the range of choice of possible particular adjustments, and the more intelligent and effective will be the neutralization of the desire.*

This principle may be seen in the typical conversation of people of different degrees of intelligence. The person whose intelligence is restricted limits his interests and conversation to particular experience, to what so-and-so said on a particular occasion ; he limits himself largely to the particular concerns of food and clothing and other more immediate considerations in his daily life. To him a conversation in terms of universals has no appeal. To him an example of a principle represents the example only. He does not take a particular as the promise of a universal. His attempts to talk the language of universals are ineffective because his attempted universals do not represent the focal statement of a normally felt need. Since the psychological act is in his mind seldom focal at the stage of universals, he cannot be expected to be very keenly aware of his limitations except as he may judge of them by the shortcomings in the consequences of his thinking. He is therefore not especially useful as an agent to resolve difficulties that have a wide range of ramifications. It is only natural that he should attain peace of mind and self-respect by claiming preference for concrete-mindedness. He is " practical ".

3. TEMPERAMENTAL ATTITUDES TOWARD INTELLECTUAL WORK

There is a general impression about the opposite type of mind that has considerable psychological interest in con-nexion with the characteristics of the reflex circuit. I am referring to the not infrequent description of profound thinkers as inactive physically, as sedentary in habits, and as lacking in the aggressiveness which is characteristic of the man of action. Not all profound thinkers are physically superior and aggressive. When such men are found, they become very soon recognized as superior men, and acknow-ledged as such by being given social responsibility of various kinds. The psychological reasonableness of this general observation may be seen if we consider it in relation to the strength of the motives and the ideo-motor tendency by which the motives tend to express themselves in action. Assume that the motives are of superior strength to corre-spond with the superior physical vitality of the man. These strong motives may be compared to high pressure in a hydraulic or an electrical analogy. When they are released to express themselves, they will exert more pressure toward the overt terminal end of the circuit than if they were relatively weak at the source. The ideo-motor tendency is the tendency of every motive to express itself in overt adjustment. This expression is, as I have previously described, a process of particularizing the motive. Now, if the ideo-motor tendency of a motive is strong, it is reasonable to expect that the motive will appear more readily towards the particularized end of the circuit than in its earlier and universal stages. If the ideo-motor tendency of a motive is relatively weak it is more apt to become focal at its loosely defined and universal stage of completion. Hence it is, in one sense, easier for a person of relatively weak impulses to be profound than for the person whose life-impulses are strong.

I have shown in a previous section that the capacity to think in terms of universals, in what we know as higher forms, implies the inhibition of the motive at its unfinished, universal, and loosely specified stage. *To think with superior intelligence is to render focal our purposes when they have acquired only the few attributes which are sufficient to point towards types of adjustment rather than specified adjustments.* This inhibition of the motive at the universal stages of the reflex circuit is, of course, more readily attained if the motive is progressing under low pressure. If the motive drives towards expression under high pressure, it is not so likely to become focal while it is still universal. It will then become focal when it is almost specified and needs only immediate perceptual guidance for its final overt completion. This should make it psychologically consistent that those men who have strong motives are frequently found to be lacking in their willingness or their ability to do analytical thinking. When the motives are relatively weak at the source they can be more readily inhibited at their early and universal stage for conceptual thinking. The general impression about profound thinkers is perhaps not so far wrong in that they are frequently men with relatively weak instinctive drives, who can for this reason render focal these drives as universals more readily than men whose instinctive drives are powerful and tend strongly towards overt expression.

These observations should not lead us to the conclusion that men of superior intellect are necessarily weaklings. We should, however, be able to admit as reasonable that the person whose life-impulses are weak finds it easier to engage in profound, analytical, abstruse reasoning than one whose life-impulses are overpoweringly strong.   The factors of mental capacity and interest must not, of course, be over-looked.   The effective man for society is no doubt the one who combines strong life-impulses with sufficient mental capacity for abstruse mental work.   He will find, however, that to him analytical work is more irksome, and it requires of him more self-control than is the case with his less vigorous brother.

The comparison that I have drawn is between two types of men who differ supposedly in the strength of their native instinctive drives.   The same kind of comparison can be made for the different strengths of two motives in the same man, or the different strengths of the same motive on different occasions.   Consider the motive to protect our physical selves.   If we know that a physical danger is to be met twelve months from now, we can render our motive of self-protection focal as a universal and consider the relative advantages of different types of adjustment in relation to the danger.   Thinking in terms of universals can then be indulged in quite readily because there is the necessary time available and the motive is not under intense pressures Consider the same situation when we are suddenly confronted with the danger to our physical selves.   If the situation at this moment is one of life and death, the pressure of the motive to express itself is intensely high, and there is no time available to debate about the relative advantages of different types of adjustment. Thinking, if there is any, is of the concrete and specific sort. Our motives are then under such intense pressure that they cannot possibly be inhibited at their universal stage of formation. They issue in the line of least resistance at the moment and in some particular form. Mental activity in such cases is of the closely specified and perceptual kind, or at most of a low order of imaginal thinking which is close to the motorium.

4. INSTINCTIVE AND RATIONAL CONDUCT

There is a continuum from instinctive conduct to rational conduct. The behaviour that we know as instinctive is typically that which becomes focal at the perceptual stage of formulation. In Fig. 4 we have a diagrammatic representation of that behaviour which we know as instinctive. It is represented by an impulse that defines itself quite suddenly and without becoming focal at its universal stages of formation. An instinctive act appears in focal consciousness in perceptual form, or in ideational form which is close to the perceptual level of definition. The instinctive act is differentiated from the ordinary perceptual or ideational impulse in that the instinctive act is more urgent; the impulse is stronger and demands an immediate expression. It is the strength of the impulse that makes it particularize itself to the perceptual level, or the closely defined ideational level, before becoming focal. Its strength is a hindrance to free trial-and-error choice or anticipation of consequences. In the diagram, the instinctive act is represented as being retarded at the perceptual level to indicate that trial-and-error choice is, in typically instinctive behaviour, ordinarily limited to the perceptual details. *Every instinctive act is conscious.* If an act is not conscious it is automatic, and it is not then strictly speaking instinctive.

Rational behaviour differs from instinctive behaviour mainly in that rational behaviour is subject to more deliberate trial-and-error choice by anticipating the consequences of overt fulfilment of the impulse. Both rational and instinctive behaviour are instinctively driven, but that conduct is said to be rational which was, before its overt expression, subject to anticipation and selection. An example will make clear the distinction. If a man has been offended by an opponent, his impulse is to dispose of the opponent. The act is instinctively driven as far as its source is concerned. The act of retaliation against the opponent may, however, be rational, or instinctive, or both. If he yields to the impulse of the moment to strike or otherwise to injure the opponent, without anticipation of consequences, or without anticipation of the expected effectiveness of the blow, his conduct is strongly instinctive. The impulse might be so strong that no counter motive of self-respect, or of social approval, would stop the impulsive expression. If, on the other hand, he stops to consider that, instead of striking his opponent impulsively at the present instant, he can effect injury in some other indirect way with more security to himself, he is to that extent rational about it. *The actions that we think of as instinctive are typically those in which the impulse is so strong that it rushes through the reflex circuit and out into overt expression with the barest perceptual guidance. Every act that is instinctive, either within man or within animals, is conscious at the perceptual stage of formation. The instinctive act is said to be rational to the extent that it is the subject of anticipation before precipitating in overt form.*

The last few paragraphs can be summarized in the principle that the ideo-motor tendency drives and particularizes the dissatisfaction toward the overt terminal end of the circuit. When this particularizing tendency is strong, the motive slides through the choice of universals by entering one of them at random. The motive appears as focal when it is almost completely defined and when it needs only final perceptual guidance. When the particularizing tendency is strong and urgent, the necessary inhibition for higher thinking, for choice among universals, is correspondingly more difficult. It is probable that this principle can be applied with profitable results not only to the differences between men, but also to the differences in the same motive as it appears in different degrees of urgency on different occasions in the same man.

The two contrasting situations that I have been describing can be thought of as graphically represented in Figs. 7 and 8. In Fig. 7 we have the motive or instinctive drive becoming focal as a relatively particularized suggestion or idea. In Fig. 8 we have a schematic representation of the motive becoming focal at a less closely defined stage, in the form of a universal. It is then a suggested policy or type of adjustment rather than a closely specified one.

5. URGENCY AND INTELLIGENCE

There are two principal factors which determine whether the motive will on any particular occasion become focal as a universal or as a particularized imaginal experience or idea. These two factors are the intelligence of the actor and the urgency or degree of dissatisfaction of the motive. These two factors work in opposite directions. The more intelligent the actor, the earlier will the dissatisfaction tend to become focal. He will tend to discuss the situation in the large with its social, scientific, financial, and other types of consequences. It is the preferred way in which his mental machinery assists him in getting out of trouble. This very capacity makes him able in many situations to adapt himself to a trouble before that trouble becomes imminent. The other factor of urgency tends to force the motive toward expression under such pressure that it does not have a chance to elaborate with conscious selection among universals. It issues suddenly under pressure at random into something definite that can be done in the emergency even though it might not be the absolutely best possible adaptive adjustment. The ideo-motor pressure can itself be analysed as dependent not only on the perceptual evidence of dissatisfaction but also on the native and normal strength of the motive which is to be expressed. Given the same situation equally perceptible to two men, such as a given case of distress, and they will act with different degrees of pressure depending on the relative strengths of their gregarious or other motives.

The two factors of urgency and intelligence as applicable to behaviour are more or less opposed. If an impulse is strong, if the demands of a situation are extremely urgent, such as the situation of getting out of a burning building, the impulse will reach overt expression without much noticeable anticipation or rational guidance. If the impulse is relatively weak, as it always is when a spatially and temporally remote benefit is being considered, the exercise of intelligence is thereby actually facilitated. This leads us to the peculiar but undoubtedly correct conclusion that if the urgency of a situation is reduced to a minimum, we can readily show our best intelligence about it. If the urgency is really very serious, we are relatively less able to use intelligence in meeting it. If these two propositions should be pushed to their logical extremes, we should have it that the condition favouring maximum intelligence is the complete absence of desire (or death) and that the conditions most urgent for life are just those in which intelligence is naturally absent. The biological function of intelligence is, of course, to be seen in its survival value for these benefits which are more or less remote in future time, either in fractional parts of a second, or in decades, as the case may be.

This interesting antithesis between urgency and intelligence can be seen in our everyday conduct and conversation. If we have nothing personally at stake in a dispute between people who are strangers to us, we are remarkably intelligent about weighing the evidence and in reaching a rational conclusion. We can be convinced in favour of either of the fighting parties on the basis of good evidence. But let the fight be our own, or let our own friends, relatives, fraternity brothers, be parties to the fight, and we lose our ability to see any other side of the issue than our own. How many of us could calmly give credit, during the war, to Germany's side of the case ? And yet we found no difficulty in listening intelligently to the pros and cons in the Russo-Japanese war. The more urgent the impulse, or the closer it comes to the maintenance of our own selves, the more difficult it becomes to be rational and intelligent. If your machine collides with another, your mind is immediately filled with all the traffic rules that favour your side of the case, and you are equally oblivious of the particular rules that favour the other man's case. Intelligence is momentarily in abeyance because the impulse of self-maintenance is at that moment too strong to be intelligent. If it were possible for a human being to be of perfect intelligence, it would be impossible for him ever to move. He would die of intelligence because he would be so deliberative that no decision could ever be made about anything.

There is another interesting difference in the situations arising from the early and the late focus in the reflex circuit. I have previously called attention to the fact that to think in terms of universals requires time and this is not available in the situations where the ideo-motor pressure is intense. This external circumstance is, however, only a reflection of a more fundamental distinction between the thinking which is in terms of particulars and that which is in terms of universals. When a man thinks in terms of universals he is usually planning not only for a future event for which he has now the leisure to plan, but he is also planning for a remote benefit, a future advantage, an advantage which is itself, more often than not, stated in terms of universals. We might put this in another way by noting that the motive which becomes focal in terms of its universals is realized as a generalized motive, a temporally remote advantage to a self which is usually more idealized than the immediate physical one. If two men are engaged in a discussion about the Federal Reserve system, they are choosing among universals, among large future types of adjustment. The self which is to gain by their possible conclusions is a more idealized self than that which usually figures in a discussion about the choices which are now before us in this perceptually defined environment. To think in terms of universals, in terms of types of adjustment, in terms of actions which are as yet only loosely organized, is to choose for a relatively remote future completion, to gain something for a universal or idealized aspect of the self.

6.   THE PRE-FOCAL IMPULSE

The previous discussion in this section may in a sense be considered as a preliminary statement for the description of what I consider to be a fundamental aspect of the preconscious part of the reflex circuit. I have divided the circuit into two main phases, namely the preconscious and the conscious. In the development of the motive toward overt expression it passes first through the elaboration of the preconscious and becomes focal in more or less specified form for final conscious guidance. The point that I shall now make clear is that the preconscious phase of the circuit does involve some particularization of the motive over which we do not have any control. When we find ourselves in a dilemma of some kind we are at first keenly conscious of the dissatisfaction in its cognitive terms. But we do not in that initial attitude have anything to suggest by which to resolve the difficulty. This is the preconscious stage of the future act by which we shall ultimately resolve the difficulty. The common expression that one is " stumped " refers to this preconscious stage of the particular adjustment which is to prove successful. But that adjustment is not yet focal even in universal form. The attitude is characteristically one of waiting. It is not infrequently accompanied by random overt expressions which are ineffective, but which nevertheless show that a strong motive is seeking expression and neutralization by some overt adjustment which has not yet been found.

When the motive does become focal it is hailed by the exclamation that " we have an idea ". When the idea occurs, it is the motive which has become partly particularized without any conscious guidance on our part We should not make the mistake of assuming that the motive is simply housed, as it were, under the cover of the preconscious and that it suddenly springs into sight, unaltered. The idea should not be divorced from the motive. The idea is not simply an associative affair ; it should be thought of as identical with the motive. In fact, the idea can be thought of as the motive which now has more clothes on, in the form of additional attributes and specifications. Stated in a crude way, we might represent the idea as equal to the motive plus attributes, sufficient to indicate the general way in which the motive proposes to express itself. Suppose that you find yourself in a somewhat strained relation with a friend. You realize the strained relation and you wish to re-establish friendly relations. This is the preconscious stage in the definition of that which you are going to do about it. You get an idea, the idea to invite him for dinner on some suitable provocation. That idea contains your purpose as its most important ingredient. Your purpose to re-establish friendly relations has now been particularized to the stage of the reflex circuit in which the motive has sufficient attributes to become focal. The motive is on its way to express itself in action. Do not think that the idea is merely associated with your purpose. The idea actually *is* your purpose which has now become more definite.

The interesting point is that *when the motive becomes focal, it has acquired attributes, the selection of which is not subject to conscious choice. This is the most outstanding difference between the preconscious and the conscious elaboration of the motive.* The later conscious particularization is subject to conscious elimination if the particulars are inconsistent with the motive. But the appearance of that which is to be particularized is almost entirely beyond our control. *Genius is the name that we give to the type of mind that more or less readily produces the idea that the rest of us can test and verify to successful overt issue.* In this sense the distinguishing mark of genius is not so much in what he consciously does as in that which he unwittingly produces out of the uncontrolled and preconscious elaboration of his purposes. The clever idea is a partly particularized dissatisfaction. When the dissatisfaction becomes completely particularized, it is an overt adjustment which is expected to neutralize the dissatisfaction. There are indirect ways in which we may attempt more or less successfully to favour the appearance of clever ideas. To worry about the problem for a time is a favourable condition for the production of clever ideas by which to solve it. To become familiar with many of the particularized expressions of related problems favours the appearance of the clever idea in that attributes are then available which might be of service. However, it is probable that great concentration on habitual expressions of the problem reduces the chances of being presented with a novel idea. Even in science there is to a certain extent a psychological antithesis between high scholarship and production. When the idea does appear it is already clothed with some attributes which were not given in the problem as it was felt. Does it not seem important that psychology should study the conditions of the preconscious elaboration of our motives and not centre all of its efforts on the later conscious verification of them ?

The last two points regarding the reflex circuit can be summarized as follows :—(1) *The preconscious part of the circuit actually accomplishes some degree of particularization of the motive,* and (2) *the preconscious particularization of the motive is beyond our control and must be patiently waited for.*

7. Precognition

I have spoken of the two phases of the reflex circuit as though they were divided by a sharp line of separation at the moment when the motive becomes focal. This is frequently a true description of what really seems to take place when the transition from the preconscious elaboration to the conscious verification is a sudden one. There are relatively frequent attitudes which can be described as transition stages between the preconscious and the conscious definition of the motive. I shall call these attitudes *precognitive* with reference to the future adjustment to which they lead. The precognitive stage of the reflex circuit is the transition stage between the preconscious and the conscious phases of it. When I say that the psychological act is precognitive at one of its stages, the reader may perhaps get the impression that I am considering as possible a moment of consciousness without cognitive elements, but that is not implied in the designation precognitive. The present moment of our conscious stream may be precognitive with reference to an adjustment that we shall make, and about which we are now concerned, but which has not yet appeared as a suggested solution or as a hopeful and possible idea. The transition stage that I am calling precognition is marked essentially by its affective aspects. It is marked by noticeable likes and dislikes for groups of cognitive terms.

Let us consider these likes and dislikes for groups of cognitive terms in the light of the particularization that takes place in the formation of the psychological act. Let us consider the state of irritation or dissatisfaction as the relatively unlocalized early part of the psychological act. The act is to become particularized, delimited to some specific adjustment, by which the irritation is to be removed and satisfaction regained. When the bright idea appears we begin to feel relieved because the need is then being specified in terms of the expected successful adjustment. But before that bright idea occurs to us, we may be having a state of delimitation of the possible courses of action. This delimitation may be a process of rough elimination of undesirable types of adjustment and a liking for certain types of adjustment. We do not yet have any definite idea as to what to do about the trouble that is now making us think. But we may have a state of mind in which we are keenly interested in certain topics of conversation, certain groups of cognitive terms, certain kinds of action, while at the same time we may have strong aversion or disgust for certain other topics of conversation or kinds of conduct. At this stage we are in reality beginning to delimit our adjustment by favouring certain things and avoiding certain other things. We may not actually be aware of the need that is causing these strong likes and dislikes. Nevertheless this attitude of mind is a significant part of the process of particularization that goes on in the formation of the psychological act. When we get the bright idea that begins to give us relief it is usually one of these favoured topics that we have defined somewhat more closely, and which is then functioning as a particularized form of the irritation in its course toward overt expression and total relief.

The stage of particularization that I have just described is what I call precognition, because it is marked by affective states of appetition and aversion for groups of cognitive terms without having reached the point at which any of these cognitive forms represents definitely a proposed resolution of the dissatisfaction. *Consciousness is of course focal in the sense that there is focal content present. But none of the focal content in the precognitive stage of the act is taken as representative of the thing that we propose to do.* The term "precognition" refers, not to that which happens to to be focal at the moment, but specifically to that which we shall eventually do in order to relieve the present state of unrest. The groups of cognitive terms which are marked by our feeling of appetition or aversion constitute what we know as complexes in the broadest interpretation of that term. The complex is in this liberal interpretation a group of cognitive terms for which we have a strong preference or avoidance. The term "complex" is used by some writers to mean special cases of this broader definition.

A very common illustration of the effect that I am here discussing is the search for a word. At the time when we are searching for the word we feel that we know what we want, but that knowledge can only be expressed at the present stage by a like or a dislike for the words that may be suggested. Certain words are felt distinctly to be closer to what we want than certain other words, and yet the right word has not yet come. This attitude of mind is precognitive with reference to the particular word that is finally to be decided upon. This illustration is a relatively trivial case of the likes and dislikes which in much stronger form, and with fundamental life motives involved, constitute what we know as complexes in the liberal interpretation of that term. The more restricted interpretation of the term would limit the complexes to the phenomena of the abnormal mind. The psychological nature of the category is the same in either case. The latter interpretation specifies the term to a more restricted range of phenomena.

Let us now shift our attention from the particularizing process as such to these groups of cognitive terms through which the particularization takes place or through which particularization is avoided. We have then several fundamental characteristics of these cognitive groups that may serve as bases for important psychological categories. In the first place the preferences and prejudices may be permanent characteristics of the personality of the actor; they may be temporary for a few days owing to local temporary circumstances, or they may be only momentary as in the search of a trivial motive for suitable expression in the course of an ordinary conversation. The groups of cognitive terms may be marked by the fact that we prefer them or avoid them. The former might be called positive complexes, and the latter might be called negative complexes, if we allow the term " complex " for both of these categories. Another line of distinction is with reference to the nature of the motive that makes its presence noticeable by these likes and dislikes. Is it a native and instinctive motive which reveals itself, or is it derived, secondary and acquired motive ? The secondary drives are probably all derived originally from the native sources, but the acquired drives seem to live a relatively independent existence when they have once been established as habitual forms of conduct. It is probable that the energy for them is in all cases tapped from the truly native instinctive sources. The distinction between native and acquired complexes is of considerable practical importance. Thus it is a native complex to show a certain kind of interest in the opposite sex while it is an acquired complex to be afraid of closed places. I shall venture the guess that the native complexes are usually positive, whereas the acquired complexes are more frequently negative, especially when they are of the abnormal sort. It is not unlikely that the sentiments may be defined in terms of the characteristics of precognition that I have here described. A prejudice would be a complex of the negative kind that has been acquired, but which is not severe enough to throw the individual socially out of balance. A typical complex of the abnormal mind would be of the negative type, driven usually by one of the main life motives directly from its source.

8. Summary

I shall summarize this section with special reference to Fig. 9. I have divided the reflex circuit into two main phases, the preconscious and the conscious. *The preconscious phase of the circuit has to do with the feeling of the problem. The conscious phase of the circuit has to do with the resolution of the problem.* As a division between these two phases of the circuit we have the moment of time when the suggested solution occurs. This moment I have referred to as the focus of the circuit. It is the moment when the resolution of the problem becomes focal. The further progress of the idea toward execution is in the nature of a particularization of the suggested idea. One must not forget that there is a process of particularization previous to the focus. The idea that occurs as a suggested resolution of a difficulty is partly particularized when it appears in the focus of consciousness. That particularization was accomplished in the preconscious phase of the circuit. *These two phases differ in one fundamental respect in that we have conscious control in elimination and selection of means to an end in the conscious part of the circuit, but we do not have any control whatever over the particularizations that take place before the suggested solution becomes focal.* Not infrequently we observe a gradual transition from the preconscious to the conscious phase of the circuit. I have called this transition phase precognition. *Precognition is the crisis of the reflex circuit.* This stage is mainly characterized by the fact that we are then in a state of preference and avoidance for large groups of cognitive terms without being able to settle on any definite term as a proposed solution of the difficulty. This stage represents a process of delimitation or particularization which is marked primarily by its affective elements although the affective elements do not at that stage exist without a cognitive core.

CHAPTER VII

OVERT AND MENTAL TRIAL AND ERROR

1. OVERT TRIAL AND ERROR

We have considered the primary function of mind to be the intermediary by which the wants of the organism become satisfied. Its basic function is the anticipation of experience, including the overt behaviour and the consequences of behaviour in the satisfactions that the organism is seeking. Consciousness is essentially the anticipation of contact experience and satisfaction in terms of the sensory cues which indicate what the expected experience is going to be like, if it is completely enacted. This equivalence enables the organism to steer its course in preparing adjustments before these adjustments are actually carried out. The development of intelligence is marked by the capacity to select among incomplete and tentative indices of conduct the ones that are to be fruitful, without actually trying these incomplete actions in final overt form.

The lowest form of mental organization, the one in which mentality is, strictly speaking, entirely absent, is that in which every impulse is carried out into behaviour without inhibition or choice. The behaviour is then entirely random. The life-impulses of the organism become automatically random behaviour, and this random behaviour is kept up until satisfaction is attained, when the motive power for the random behaviour disappears and the random restless behaviour ceases. This is what we shall call overt trial and error. The point at which the trial-and-error choices are made is at the terminal end of the circuit. Think of a cat trying to get out of a box without knowing how to operate the latch of the door. Here we have a motive to get out of the box. The motive would normally issue by simply stepping out. Since this does not work, the motive defines itself by random expression, pawing, scratching, and pushing. The motive is to be thought of as a pressure or force that expresses itself in various ways, more or less at random, until the motive suddenly is neutralized and disappears. The particular move that satisfies the motive is said to be the successful one. It is arrived at by random trial and error. Each move is actually executed without noticeable anticipation of consequences. Each failure is objectively recorded in the environment and in time.

2. Perceptual Trial and Error

The primary function of the sense-organs is to enable the organism to deal with incomplete behaviour, to select among tentative actions before they are completely expressed. The tentative actions are represented by the sense-impressions. It is clear that the distance sense departments afford a control over future action more effectively than the control that is possible by the contact sense-impressions. The visual sense-impression is in effect an index of expected action. Its effectiveness as a means for perceptual trial-and-error choice depends on the fact that in the past history of the organism the visual impression and the contact experience have been experienced together. The visual impression normally precedes the contact experience and hence, on subsequent occasions, the visual impression alone serves to select the action which would finally be taken if the contact experience were allowed to complete itself.

If we think of ourselves in the situation of the cat that is trying to escape from a box, we would discover fewer random overt acts if the urgency of the situation were not too strong. We would look at the walls of the box, and if they are found by their visual appearance to be flimsily constructed, we might push through the wall to freedom. If, on the other hand, the visual cue represents the wall to be made of solid brick, or iron bars, we would not so readily attempt the overt completion of the act by simply pushing ourselves through the wall. The trial-and-error choice would be made at the incomplete stage of formation at which the expected action is only a visual index of the expected contact experience. If we found a latch on the door we should have some random movements with the latch and some attitudes of visual inspection of the latch. Some of the ideas regarding the manipulation of the latch would be discarded before ever reaching overt expression. The difference between these two extremes is that in one case the random ideas that occur are executed in overt form, whereas in the second case the random ideas are checked long enough to be lived through mentally before being allowed to express themselves in overt adjustment. Both procedures illustrate trial and error. One is overt trial and error while the second is mental trial and error. All thinking is in this sense trial and error which is carried on mentally instead of overtly. The intelligent adjustment is one that is executed only after having been anticipated mentally.

3. Perception as a Conditioning Process

The behaviouristic school of psychology has as one of its fundamental experimental procedures the conditioning process. If a pain stimulus is given to an animal simultaneously with the ringing of a bell, and if this coincidence is repeated a number of times, it is found that the ringings of the bell alone will elicit the same reaction of withdrawal as the normal pain stimulus. The auditory stimulus has then been grafted, as it were, on the reaction which is normally made to the pain stimulus. The reaction to pain can, by such experimental methods, be obtained from the auditory stimulus in the absence of the pain stimulus by the mere fact that the two stimuli have been closely associated on a number of occasions. This is known as the process of conditioning.

This process of conditioning is, by no means, a special phenomenon. It is basic for the very process of perception itself. The visual impressions of a knife are associated with the contact experience of handling it and using it. The visual reflections from the smooth steel surface are associated with smoothness to the touch. The appearance of the knife and of the edge are associated with the relative ease or difficulty of cutting with the knife. After a number of such experiences the visual impressions alone, without the associated contact experience, serve the same purpose as the combination of the visual and the contact experiences. The visual sense-impression has then acquired meaning in the true sense of the word. The action of using the knife is then facilitated or inhibited in terms of the incomplete form of it which is the visual sense-impression alone. We have then profited by experience. We have learned. We are then able to remove the trial-and-error process from the realm of overt behaviour to the stage at which the behaviour is still incomplete and mental. If it were not for this conditioning process, perception and mentality would have no biological function.

4. IDEATIONAL TRIAL AND ERROR

We have described the trial-and-error process as taking place either in overt form or in the form of incomplete mental antecedents of action. By perceptual trial and error we mean the process of selecting from among those perceived possibilities of behaviour that one which means the desired consequences in terms of past identity of the sense-experience and the corresponding contact experience. The impulse may appear in the degree of definition which corresponds to the percept with the exception that the stimulus or sensory cue has not yet been found. When that happens we have ideational trial and error. The impulse is facilitated or it fails to remain identified with the momentary self in accordance with its degree of similarity with the impulses that constitute the self at the moment. If an impulse particularizes itself in such a way that it becomes more and more unlike the desires that constitute the self, there is a corresponding reduction in the urgency or reality of the impulse. If it defines itself with particulars that frustrate the motives of the self, the impulse disappears altogether. The impulse, it must be remembered, is not something apart from the self. The self is made up of these impulses, and they remain vital and urgent factors in determining behaviour only in so far as they retain their identity with the inner self as they complete themselves toward action. The process of adding attributes to the impulse in its course toward expression is entirely fortuitous as far as the self is concerned. It depends largely on the past experience of the actor and on the flexibility of his mentality. He has himself no control over the particularized forms that his impulses will take. *The self consists in the impulses in their universal unlocalized form. The detailed expressions of the impulses do not necessarily represent the true self.*

Suppose that an executive is considering the relative advantages of two policies such as promotion to positions of responsibility from within the organization and the selection of outsiders for such positions. The former alternative makes for good morale by placing before the employees an objective. The second alternative gives the opportunity to bring in new talent and the advantage of a wide field in which to choose trained men. To make up one's mind on such a problem is to state the problem in its abstract form, in the form of a policy, and to let this particularize itself in as many ways as possible.

In Fig. 10 we have a diagrammatic representation of the intension-extension attributes of impulses at different stages of the reflex circuit. If an impulse is being the subject of trial-and-error choice while it is still in the form of a universal, there are many variations of behaviour that are possible as detailed expressions of the impulse. If, on the other hand, the impulse does not become focal for trial-and-error choice until it has defined itself closely, there are, of course, only a relatively small number of possible variations in behaviour among which to specify the impulse into conduct. If the impulse be focal for conscious selection at the stage D there would be, in the diagram, twice as many forms of possible behaviour as

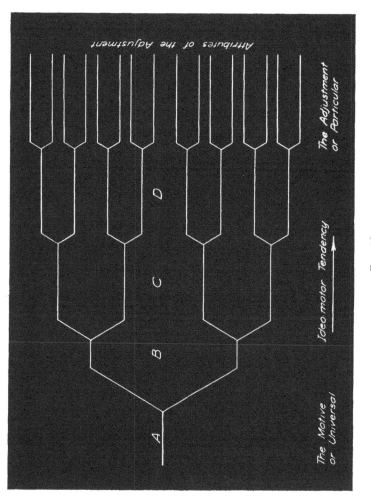

Attributes of the Adjustment

The Adjustment
or Particular

Ideo-motor Tendency

The Motive
or Universal

A   B   C   D

Fig. 10.

[To face p. 118.

if the impulse is not conscious until it reaches overt expression in the form of its consequences. If the impulse is rendered focal at the stage B while still a loosely organized universal or concept, there are eight times as many lines of behaviour possible as in overt trial and error. Each of the eight actions may be anticipated mentally and eliminated if they prove to be failures without ever recording the failures on the environment. The numerical relations of the diagram are of course entirely arbitrary for illustrative purposes.

If a boy is asked to construct the arc of a circle of three inches radius so that it will be tangent to two given circles, he may proceed with several degrees of intelligence. He may proceed by the cat's method, sticking the compass into the drawing aimlessly and drawing circles with centres and radii entirely at random until the task is done. This would be overt trial and error without conscious guidance All the failures would be objectively recorded on the environment and none of them would be mentally inhibited.

He might proceed with the degree of intelligence that ordinary vision affords. He would then foresee the absurdity of some of his previous circles, and these absurdities would be abandoned mentally without being recorded on his environment. This would be an example of perceptual intelligence.

He might notice the inevitable common element of the three-inch radius in all successful adjustments and set his compass accordingly for all his trials. This would be an abstraction in that his problem is made focal at an unfinished stage. He would still make several errors before locating the right centre. If he were to strip the problem of all the details that are not necessary to identify it, he would be dealing with the principles of constructive geometry, and he would locate the correct centre without recording any failures on the drawing. That would be ideational or conceptual intelligence. His trial-and-error process would be taking place with impulses to draw circles while these impulses were still only principles of geometry instead of actual muscular movements with the compass in hand.

5. Conceptual Trial and Error

I recently heard a discussion of the policies of the League of Nations. The particular topic was the nature of the police power by which the League should maintain its decisions. It was suggested that the League should enforce its decisions by public opinion in all the nations of the League. This was presented as a novel idea because we have hitherto always taken for granted that the two items " court " and " police " are necessary attributes of law and order. The novelty of the proposed solution consists psychologically in that its author stripped the item " police " as a superfluous attribute from his concept of civic order. He allowed his concept to particularize itself along some other route toward practical execution. This route can be represented as a cross-road that bears the sign " international public opinion ". This sign we are now stopping to look at. The road that we have always taken in the past bears the sign " military police power ", but we have been so accustomed to take this

road that we have never even seen the sign. Both roads
are expressions of the motive to have civic order. We have
never before been conscious at so early and abstract a stage
in the expression of this motive. We are in the habit of
adding preconsciously the attributes of military police power
so that these attributes are already present and taken for
granted when the motive becomes focal for conscious
selection of further particulars.

We can represent the pre-focal particularization as though
we were passing a fork in the road at night while we are
asleep. In the morning we wake up and are consulted
about the cross-roads further on. The cross-roads that
we passed during the night are taken for granted because
we know nothing about them. The later cross-roads are,
of course, of more restricted significance than the choices
that could have been made earlier in the trip. The decision
at every fork in the road represents the addition of particulars
to the motive in its course toward overt expression. Our
location when we wake up represents the status of the
motive when it becomes focal. The turns that are made
after we wake up represent the control of foresight or
intelligence. At every turn we attempt to live through
imaginally what we may expect ahead of us. We inhibit
our progress until we have done this, and we make our
choice, if it is done rationally, on the basis of such mental
trial and error. The maximum control and foresight
and the widest range of possible adjustment is in general
attained by the individual who can make focal his motives
in their skeletal and abstract form before they have absorbed
any habitual or preconsciously preferred attributes. The

thinker is the man who does not take for granted even that which is generally accepted as common sense. Even our habitual ways of doing things and our preconscious preferences are evaluated by him as though they were possible alternatives, but by no means as though they were the inevitable and only ones.

I have in this section shown the application of the various principles of intelligent adjustment that I have so far discussed. I have assumed a universal ideo-motor tendency for all conscious life. It is not sufficient to say that ideas tend sooner or later to express themselves in action. Ideas always tend to define themselves motorially. The effect of this universal tendency on the psychological object I have called particularization. Intelligent conduct implies the inhibition of a motive at an undefined stage in order to make it focal in its incomplete form. By so doing we are better able to select its further particulars and eliminate mentally lived failures from overt expression. This has also been described as essentially a process of trial and error which takes place mentally instead of overtly with consequent survival value for the organism. All conscious life is according to this point of view to be considered as unfinished action, and its biological value is to be judged in the light of the adaptive adjustments to which the conscious operations actually lead. Finally, an abstraction is an unfinished want or need which is focal for the purpose of selecting with foresight the means of neutralizing it. An abstraction of a high order is, accordingly, a want which is focal when it has only a relatively small number of attributes. To think is to test the tentative additional attributes by living their consequences imaginally.

CHAPTER VIII

Suppose that the motive on a particular occasion is to resolve a difficulty for which one would ordinarily think of money as the solution. The motive can define itself in any one of many different particular forms such as to borrow the money from a friend, at the bank, earn it, delay some other payment, give a note, charge it, and so on. Suppose that the motive defines itself in the idea of borrowing the money from a friend. Additional attributes are necessary in the form of deciding from whom to borrow.

At each step in this process of particularization the motive discards all but one of the several possibilities until it issues in overt form. Now suppose that the motive to get some money for an emergency is allowed to issue impulsively and without conscious selection at the successive stages. It may then issue as a request of a friend who happens to be near just at this moment. It might be an inopportune moment, and it might be the wrong friend. The overt expression of the motive results in failure, i.e. the motive is not neutralized and its pressure is still felt. We may formulate this unintelligent particularization as follows :—

1. Emergency
2. Emergency+money
3. Emergency+money+borrow it
4. Emergency+money+borrow it+of a friend
5. Emergency+money+borrow it+of a friend+this friend
6. Emergency+money+borrow it+of a friend+this friend+right now

The particularization is unintelligently said and done, and it results in failure. The above definition of the motive follows the line of least resistance without inhibition, foresight, or conscious choice of means to an end.

Now suppose that we introduce a modicum of intelligence into this adjustment. This would consist of an inhibition of a late stage of the motive as, for example, at step number 5. You are going to ask this particular friend for the money but you anticipate the embarrassment of fulfilling your motive right now while he is talking with a group of people. You decide to approach him during the course of the evening. The motive has been allowed to express itself by following the line of least resistance, by impulsive and unconscious particularization to the perceptual stage. Conscious guidance appears first only as you are about to step over to this friend with your errand. Then you foresee the consequence and inhibit. You allow the motive, as it appears at 5, to particularize itself again along some other route—such as asking this friend later in the evening. If that is not inconsistent with your various motives such as getting the money and your desire for social approval, the motive will express itself overtly in this way.

Let us now introduce more intelligence into this adjustment. Instead of taking for granted impulsively that the money is to be obtained from this particular friend, we " stop " to consider. Perhaps some other friend would be a better expression of the motive. Here you will notice that the motive becomes conscious at a less defined stage such as at step 4. In the previous case we allowed the motive impulsively to pass by the stage at which some other friend might have been selected. The earlier in the psychological act we introduce conscious choice of particulars, the more intelligent is the adjustment, the fewer will be the objectively recorded failures, and the greater will be the number of available solutions which are not thought of in unintelligent and impulsive conduct.

We shall now consider a still more intelligent adjustment. Assume that the motive to get some money is inhibited at step 3. The idea is then to get out of the emergency by getting some money which we propose to borrow. At this point we stop the impulse and ask " where ? " We can particularize this impulse along several routes such as a friend, or the bank. We live mentally each of the routes that may appear, and our motive expresses itself along that course of action which is least inconsistent with the action patterns that characterize our personality. By stopping the impulse at this stage we may come upon a type of solution which would be entirely missed if we allowed the impulse to become more defined before giving conscious aid. The first requisite for the appearance of an idea is to stop and wait for it to appear. The clever idea may or may not appear depending partly on our mentality, the incentives, and the amount of thought that we have given to the problem ; but to inhibit the impulse and to wait for a new idea will at least give that new idea a chance to become focal.

If the motive is arrested at step 2 for rational guidance, we shall not be taking it for granted that the money is to be borrowed. There are other ways of getting money besides borrowing it. I am not here implying that borrowing is necessarily an unintelligent thing to do. What I am interested to show is that the impulsive and unintelligent satisfaction of a want takes for granted any solution which seems handy, and fails to discover the possible solutions which might have appeared by stating the motive in its most abstract and generalized form.   If the money-getting motive were in a still more abstract form as step 1, we should not even take for granted that money is necessary.   If the emergency is realized in the most abstract way possible we may think of some clever manœuvre which solves the difficulty without money.   The less intelligent conduct would assume many of these particulars and would represent the problem already filled with specifications that are taken for granted.   The result is that unintelligent behaviour controls only a limited range of possible adjustments.

Consider again the situation of retaliation for an insult. The pressure of an instinctive adjustment usually causes the motive to define itself through the ideational stages without rational choice of means.   The motive becomes conscious at the perceptual stage in aiming the fist.   If the motive were inhibited at a less defined stage we should have it in the form of an idea to injure our opponent—just how ?— that is what we are now thinking about.   We might discover ways of damaging his business or reputation which would in the long run be satisfactory and less dangerous for us physically.   But it is characteristic of typically instinctive behaviour that it is driven by considerable emotional pressure, and it is therefore especially difficult to inhibit the instinctive motive at an abstract or imaginal stage of completion.   For this reason it is not so often accomplished. When it is accomplished, we speak of it as a feat of self-control. I believe that instinctive and rational conduct are by no means mutually exclusive. An instinctive act is also rational if it has been defined by conscious choice of means to an end at the imaginal level of its expression.

Intelligence can in this sense be defined as a capacity which can be considered as superimposed on the ideo-motor tendency. Try to entertain the concept "lamp" for example. It tends to define itself as a particular lamp—a floor lamp—tungsten—silk shade—blue shade—it is lit—it is here—and so on. It requires inhibition of no mean order to retain a concept as such, unless we are aided by habitual manipulation of its properties, such as in mathematics or language. The same applies to sensation. It is after all quite a feat to be conscious of the sensation red without letting it become a red something.

The cortex has been described by neurologists as having for one of its functions the inhibition of the lower centres. If this is so, it is not inconsistent with the assertions here made concerning the close relationship between inhibition and intelligence, but such correspondence is only incidental if it does exist. Psychology is concerned with mental life, and it is only incidentally curious about its neurological equivalents.

CHAPTER IX

The Sense Qualities

Let us consider the fact that the energy of the stimulation of a receptor is not sufficient to account for the gross bodily adjustments of the organism. This fact makes it necessary to distinguish between two energy systems, one arising from the external stimulus and one with its source in the organism itself. These two energy systems should not be considered as hypothetical. Their existence is obvious in the fact that the amount of energy in the stimulus is insufficient to account for the bodily adjustments of the organism. These two systems are distinguished in several fundamental ways. The external system is insignificant in comparison with the internal system as far as the energy impinging on the receptor surface is concerned. The external system is fortuitous in its direction because its presence or absence to the organism depends largely on the direction in which the receptor surfaces happen to be exposed. The internal system is directed purposively for the needs and comforts of the organism as these may be realized at the moment. That cannot be said about the stimulus energy as such. These statements refer to the exteroceptors.

The interoceptors get their stimulation from the physiological conditions of the body and may be considered as serving the same rôle for the cerebro-spinal system as that served by the exteroceptors. Both the exteroceptors and the interoceptors give the cues for the cerebro-spinal machinery to be set in motion to bring about relief, and to satisfy the bodily needs.

If the stimulation touches one of the fundamental motives of the organism it will be keenly concerned and intensely conscious. The vitality of the organism supplies the energy necessary for making the gross adjustments in terms of the stimulation. It is in this sense that the stimulation acts like a trigger. The stimulation constitutes a minor energy system which releases the major internal energy sources of the organism to satisfy its wants. If the stimulation does not touch one of these internal desires, nothing happens, and the stimulation is treated with indifference. It is for this reason that our reaction to a stimulation cannot possibly be stated wholly in terms of the stimulus. The main factors determining the response are the internal conditions of the organism itself. Of course we can say that, other things being equal, a large stimulus, a moving stimulus, an intense stimulus, will attract our attention more readily than a small one, a still one, a weak one. This is on the principle that, other things being equal, the large, moving, strong, and novel stimulation is likely to indicate future discomfort, failure, and even death. But other things are not equal except in the indifferent laboratory situation. It is true that we tend to remember the last few items in a list of nonsense syllables more readily than the items in the middle of the list. But our recall is determined far more by the consideration as to whether we care about the syllables. It is possible, then, to describe the reaction as a function of the stimulation to a limited extent, if we make the assumption that the motivation is constant.

This reasoning applies readily enough to those situations in which we have a more or less conscious purpose immediately in mind. But it does not so obviously apply to those situations in which we relax and simply allow a sense-impression to register with an attitude of indifference on our part. Suppose that I am at this moment entirely calm and satisfied and that my mind is a more or less peaceful blank. I have no momentary purposes and I let my eyes turn more or less at random. Let us suppose that they fall on a glass paper-weight in front of me. I am conscious of the sense-impressions of reflected light from the glass cube. I have previously said that every conscious moment is an unfinished act, and this is true whenever consciousness serves its biological function. But in this case I am entertaining a conscious state, and I am sure that I have no purpose or action in mind. The sense-impressions are focal and yet no action is in sight or even intended. I prefer to consider these volitionally indifferent mental states as slight ripples of the internal energy system caused by the stimulation of a receptor surface. If the internal energy system, the degree of satisfaction of my various purposes at this moment, is in a state of equilibrium, it is still possible that the energy of the stimulation of a receptor may cause a slight disturbance of my internal calm. But if the stimulation is rather indifferent to my various motives, nothing will happen beyond the superficial ripple of awareness of the sense-impression. If the light which is being reflected from the paper-weight should be sufficiently intense to make me uncomfortable, the stimulation would no longer be an indifferent ripple in consciousness because it would then constitute the cue in terms of which I would make some appropriate arm and hand movement to move the paperweight so as to regain comfort. The difference between these two situations is simply that when the stimulation is indifferent to my momentary purposes, it causes only what I have called a superficial ripple in consciousness. Such a slight disturbance from an indifferent external source constitutes sensory consciousness. It is in that state that we can discriminate between sense qualities. But when the stimulation touches one of our states of satisfaction we lend from our vitality the energy to attain satisfaction in terms of the sensory cue. It is in that case that the sensory cue is lived imaginally to its equivalent contact experience. It is then that perception serves in the rôle which is its normal biological justification.

I can well imagine a sincere objection to my analysis of mental life, which would run like this : " I am not so sure that my mental states are always unfinished actions. It is not entirely obvious that my purposes always start my thinking. The stimulus seems to serve as the starting-point for my conscious state right now when I am perceiving this indifferent object." I am granting that the stimulation from the environment may be primarily responsible for 'a state of awareness. But I am considering a mere mental state of awareness as biologically insignificant and only incidental to those more important situations in which the stimulation taps one of our purposes. When the stimulation leads to an adjustment, the stimulus serves merely as a trigger to release the expression of my own purposes, the expression of my own larger energy supply. It is only that kind of stimulation which is useful for us. Indifferent awareness of sense qualities has no survival value. It is incidental to the situations in which the awareness of sense qualities serves a purpose. It is our capacity to particularize the sense-impressions to their equivalent expected contact experience, capacity to define our purposes in the form of expected experience even in the absence of the stimulation that constitutes intelligence. Purposeless awareness should be considered as a superficial ripple on consciousness, a moment of introversion, a slight disturbance caused by the action of the receptor, a trigger action which fails to release any motivation to act. If we should honestly note our sense-impressions during the course of a day we should probably find that the great majority of our percepts are actually looked for. It is relatively rare that a stimulus is not actually more or less consciously hunted for.

The sense qualities have received perhaps more attention from psychologists than any other psychological subject. If we study these sense qualities for the ultimate object of relating them to the functions of the organism as a biological unit, the study will be fruitful. This is in fact being done when sense-impressions are studied as means for space localization. As psychologists we are justified in being interested in sense qualities as such. We should not be impatient, however, with the general student who comes to us for instruction in psychology, to learn how the human mind works when it is actually working, to learn why people think, act, and live as they do. He is legitimately interested in motivation psychology. We should not expect him to be interested in the dynamically indifferent sense qualities as such. And yet we often devote the first and major part of our courses to this psychologically remote topic.

The ideal course in psychology for the beginning college student would be one in which the various human wants and desires are described as sources of conduct. These sources, in our present state of knowledge, would have to be described in terms of the types of behaviour and in terms of the types of satisfaction which they crave. It would not be necessary to insist that the description of these sources of conduct be entirely complete, or that the classifications be mutually exclusive. The main purpose should be to familiarize the student in an explicit way with what he already knows intuitively—the mainsprings of human conduct. It would do no harm to analyse the possible motives, conscious and unconscious, that may be exemplified in history, politics, the courts, literature, and biography. Complete agreement as to the sources and motives of conduct cannot be expected, but with continued study directed toward the sources of human conduct, experimental procedures for verification of hypotheses will eventually be forthcoming. What we need first of all is a shift of emphasis, a shift in the direction in which we look for explanatory categories in psychology, a shift from the mere description of the objective environment to a description of the individual himself and the satisfactions that seem to constitute his happiness. Merely to accomplish such a shift of interest in psychological teaching will immediately make it truly a study of the human mind. The quantitative point of view need not be discarded as the ideal scientific method, but its introduction into psychology has been forced to such an extent that we have found it necessary to leave mind in order to be quantitative. We have turned our attention to the measurable environment for the mere sake of being scientific and quantitative. It is more important for us to retain our true subject-matter, the human mind, even with pseudo-scientific methods, than to desert our subject-matter in order to be quantitatively scientific.

After the student has surveyed the field of human motives, he will be interested to see what happens to these motives when their expression is facilitated, frustrated, or inhibited. He will be interested to see how the human animal acts when several parallel motives clash for control, how motives seek substitute satisfactions, and how these substitute satisfactions can be consciously controlled by the individual himself and by public opinion. Then, for the student who specializes in psychology, further opportunity should be given to study the sense organs in detail and the physiological and neurological effects which are known to parallel the mental phenomena which are central for psychology.

CHAPTER X

AUTISTIC THINKING

Stated in a condensed way we should consider thinking as realistic when it looks toward actual execution in the real world about us, whereas autistic thinking is that which we indulge in for partial satisfaction of our ambitions, without intending to execute these ambitions in any real sense. If we are day-dreaming of the success that we should like to have, or of the satisfaction of our various desires, we are doing autistic thinking. If our thinking is considering the ways and means of attaining our ambitions in reality, then we are doing realistic thinking. It will of course readily be seen that there is no sharp line of distinction between these two types of thinking, although we can readily recognize the two extremes as such. This continuum from one psychological category to another is almost universal. We have previously seen this with regard to such categories as perception and imagination. The terms are useful in distinguishing types of mental activity even though they shade into each other and are inapplicable in any definite way to many ordinary mental states which involve elements of both the contrasting classifications.

The provocation for autistic thinking is found in the ease with which *mental* satisfaction of our ambitions and desires can be attained, as compared with the difficulties and the competition which are to be overcome in order actually to attain our ends. If the difficulties that confront us in the attainment of our ambitions seem almost insurmountable, there is the possibility of gaining at least momentary satisfaction by day-dreaming of success. If a person is relatively unpopular with the opposite sex, there is a kind of partial satisfaction in day-dreaming the attainment of that popularity. The weakling frequently day-dreams of feats of remarkable strength and of the admiration which he would like to enjoy but which he is either too lazy or too crippled physically to attain. The child may dream about an orgy of cake, candy, and jam, which may be partially denied in reality. We should not jump to the conclusion that all day-dreaming and all sleep-dreaming are necessarily wish-fulfilment, but that this factor is apparent in most forms of day-dreaming would probably be admitted by every frank observer of his own mental life.

Most of the psycho-analytic interpretations of mental states reduce them to expressions of wishes. The Freudian psychology is based primarily on the interpretation of free moving thought as wish-fulfilment. With this point our present discussion is entirely in accord. What we have been calling the life-impulses, the dynamic self, is identical with the libido of the psycho-analytic schools. In their writing, the origin of mental life is either explicitly stated to be in the organism, or the discussion implies such an assumption. All the environmental factors are interpreted as opportunities for the expression of the libido.

The general provocation for autistic thinking is the ease with which imaginal satisfaction of a motive may be attained compared with the usual difficulties of attaining a motive which has been sufficiently blocked to become keenly conscious. There are several typical situations under this general head which it may be profitable to keep in mind when attempting to classify any particular occurrence of autistic thinking. I shall list four such sub-classes which I should consider as logical possibilities, but I cannot say anything regarding the relative frequency of these different types of provocation for autistic thinking or day-dreaming. The first that comes to mind is that of indolence. It is conceivable that a person may have the ability to attain his ends, and that the situation is suitable and even immediately present, but that he is too indolent to act. In such a case one should probably say that the motive is, in this man, not very strong, or that he is rather unusual in some aspect of his volitional make-up.

A more interesting case would be the situation in which a man has actually tried to attain his purpose and has failed. He may then withdraw to himself, as it were, and day-dream the attainment of his ambitions instead of trying repeatedly to realize them in the environment. He may perhaps become gloomy and pessimistic. He withdraws from social contact at least in those particulars in which his frustrated motive is involved. He spends his time gaining some partial satisfaction in dreaming of the attainment of his ends and the consequences of such attainment. This situation can be thought of as rather momentary, temporary, or as a more or less permanent mental state, following a failure. Examples of the momentary kind of autistic thinking is the situation of a small boy who has been " licked " by his stronger or more dexterous opponent. The boy will imagine himself a giant, a hero, subduing his opponent with the greatest ease and receiving popular acclamation for his superiority. This illustrates a function of autistic thinking in relieving the motive partially at least in an overtly ineffectual way. I should represent this second type of autistic thinking in Fig. 11 by the motive which becomes focal at F in the thought of beating the opponent. It expresses itself overtly by the particularization A to D, as in the diagram. Suppose now that the final overt particularization of the motive in the attributes $ABCD$ fails to relieve the motive. The motive to be master is still there and it may issue in continuing the fight or it may issue merely in mental form. When the motive becomes focal, as at F, the successful overt issue is inhibited and a mental particularization of the success is substituted, as at d'. It is characteristic of autistic thinking that it is not very consistent as to the means whereby the end is to be attained. This I have indicated by leaving out of autistic thinking the plausible means whereby the end might be attained such as the particularization ABC. Autistic thinking revolves about the end D and ignores as far as possible the absence of suitable means to arrive at D. In the case of autistic thinking that we have just described we have an ineffective mental anticipation of satisfaction following an overt failure. This is another instance of the trial-and-error expression of the motive which refuses to be assimilated elsewhere immediately. Its repeated overt expression is inhibited because of its impossibility, and some partial satisfaction is gained by imagining the success which has in reality been denied.

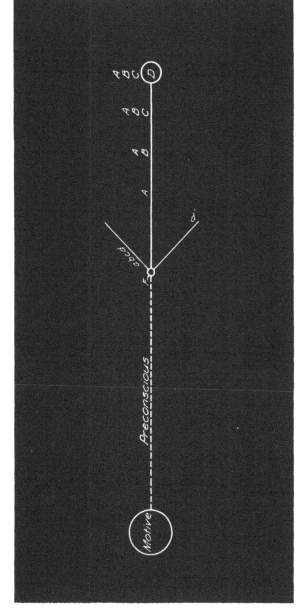

Fig. 11.

A third type of autistic thinking is caused by a motive that is too weak to force its way to successful expression in overt behaviour, especially if some resistance or inconvenience is encountered.   The motive may, nevertheless, be strong enough to cause day-dreaming.   The weak motive which expresses itself in autistic form may be indicative of a personality in which the life-impulses of various types are weak, and it may also be indicative of a personality that has not become accustomed to overcome real difficulties and to take the necessity for effort as a matter of course.   The former cause is in the weak personality itself, and the latter cause is primarily in the moral experience of the subject.

A fourth type of provocation for autistic thinking is the conflict of several motives which are simultaneously pressing for expression.   When the satisfaction of one of these motives means the frustrating of another motive, the conflict is identical with a failure which is anticipated mentally.   If the two motives are very unequal in strength, the stronger will survive and reach expression with a slight disappointment of the weaker motive.   In such cases we have mixed satisfaction, one strong motive being satisfied and a weaker motive becoming conscious as having been denied.   When both of the motives are strong we have several kinds of resolution possible.   Some of the ways in which a conflict of motives is resolved lead to insanity.

The main difference between autistic thinking and realistic thinking is not in the actual content of the thought itself, but in the attitude of the thinker toward the attainment or satisfaction for which the thinking is normally a preparation. *In realistic thinking the actor anticipates the satisfaction.   In autistic thinking the actor lives imaginally the satisfaction itself.   In realistic thinking the actor is striving to attain, whereas in autistic thinking the actor lives the attainment imaginally as though it had already been reached.*   It is not possible to differentiate the two forms of thinking merely by the content.   Both deal with imaginally represented experience.   Both deal with ideational or conceptual representations of expected experience.   Both represent a willingness of the thinker to live the imaginal experience in reality if it were readily at hand.   Both may have the appearance of abstraction, and both forms of thought may give enjoyment to the thinker.   The autistic form of thought is, of course, less critical of the means for attaining the imaginal experience because in this form of thought the instinctive satisfactions of the day-dream are represented as having already been attained.

If one is thinking about something that has no immediate behaviouristic equivalent, such as the solution of a puzzle, the satisfaction that one is seeking may be merely the feeling of control and mastery.   While thinking about the puzzle, the attitude is characteristically that of realistic thought because it is an attitude of expectation of future attainment ; it is a search with effort for the means of attaining future satisfaction ;   it is an attitude in which the ineffective spontaneous ideas are promptly discarded as soon as their ineffectiveness is definitely anticipated.   It is not, therefore, the exclusively mental reference of the thought that constitutes the criterion of autistic thinking.   The way to determine whether thinking at any moment is realistic or autistic is to ask what the attitude is with regard to attainment.   If the attainment is imaginally represented as having been reached, if the attainment is imaginally being enjoyed, the thinking can be declared with certainty to be autistic.

I have described autistic thinking as though it were entirely bad and to be shunned. Such a recommendation should be guided by the circumstances. A child that spends much time day-dreaming should be encouraged to participate in activities which involve concrete reality in order to establish as habitual a willingness to check day-dreaming occasionally with reference to its probable successful issue. But to insist on this can also be overdone. The person who lives in particulars, in concrete reality, in that which is obviously practical on the face of it, is living a life of narrow usefulness. Most concrete-minded persons who pride themselves on being " practical " live such lives. Their usefulness is necessarily restricted because their minds work exclusively with the so-called practical particulars.

It is a question of considerable practical and educational importance to determine the extent to which autistic thinking is to be encouraged or discouraged. Fundamentally, autistic thinking is not effective in reaching the solution to a pressing problem, because the thinker takes the attitude of enjoying the imaginal goal instead of devoting himself to the search for ways of attaining it in reality. But, on the other hand, we must not forget that a certain amount of the free moving thought of the autistic sort gives opportunity for many ideas to appear which would not appear with the strictly realistic process. The reason for this is that in autistic thinking there is a marked reduction in the critical evaluation of means to ends, and ideas which are remotely relevant might be discarded in the realistic attitude on account of superficial incongruity. An idea which appears in the autistic attitude may be favoured for no explicit reason but simply because it seems attractive. Such an idea is not infrequently loaded with some characteristic that is essential for an effective solution of a problem.

It is probably true that the best ideas regarding our problems come to us in attitudes that are relatively free from immediate purposive restrictions. The best thinkers are those who allow themselves a considerable amount of day-dreaming, but the interests that guide such reverie should be social in their benefits rather than individual and immediately personal. A good personality cannot be developed in the person who limits his conscious life strictly to purposive thought. When the autistic attitude is carried to extremes the actor becomes relatively useless because he evades by his autistic habits the trial-and-error struggle for attaining desired reality. Teachers should recognize the advantages and the disadvantages of autistic thinking. They should encourage it where it is entirely lacking, while discouraging it where the attitude is interfering with productive accomplishment.

CHAPTER XI

The Function of Ineffective Adjustments

There are many interesting effects in normal or momentarily disrupted mental life which may be considered under the title of this section. Let us consider a motive or dissatisfaction which is attempting to get relief through overt adjustment of some kind. The motive may be considered as a pressure which expresses itself, more or less, at random in different overt forms until one act is executed which gives relief. This drains the motive and there is no further cause for continued trial-and-error behaviour. The last act, which drained the motive and satisfied it, is called the successful act. We have in a previous section considered the manner in which the consequences of a proposed adjustment are anticipated mentally. If that anticipation is a failure the intended act is no longer driven by the motive. It is no longer identical or integral with the motive, and it therefore simply disappears. The pressure still remains and expresses itself in some other idea or anticipated act which is driven by the motive as long as the proposed act is identical with the motive. This trial-and-error process may be maintained in overt behaviour, in perceptual anticipation, or in the form of the still earlier anticipation of imagination.

Consider now the situation in which a strong motive, which is close to the mainsprings of our lives, remains unsatisfied for some time. This drive may either be dissipated by being drained into other more or less equivalent channels, or it may remain as a pressure which is ready to particularize itself in any manner through the slightest provocation. This we have also considered in relation to the sensitiveness to slights of a person who does not feel socially, professionally, financially or otherwise sure of himself. Such a person has the universal motive of self-expansion or self-assertion which has not been given adequate expression and relief.

The kind of relief to which we have so far given our attention is that which is effective, that which satisfies the motive and drains it. After its satisfaction the individual is not so sensitive to slights, perhaps, as he was before receiving something in the way of social approval and recognition unless he has lived for a long time in a submissive attitude. There are situations in which we can see a motive expressing itself overtly in ways which are entirely inadequate and totally ineffective. These constitute one of the most interesting topics in human psychology because one can study them in everyday life in oneself and in other people. They constitute good indices of the mental life and character of people, and their understanding can only be of advantage in the improvement of one's own character.

In Fig. 12 I have represented what may be thought of as taking place when a motive suddenly bursts out in an adjustment which is on some occasions absolutely detrimental to its genuine satisfaction. How does this come about ? In the diagram I have represented the motive which tends to particularize itself, to express itself. This is

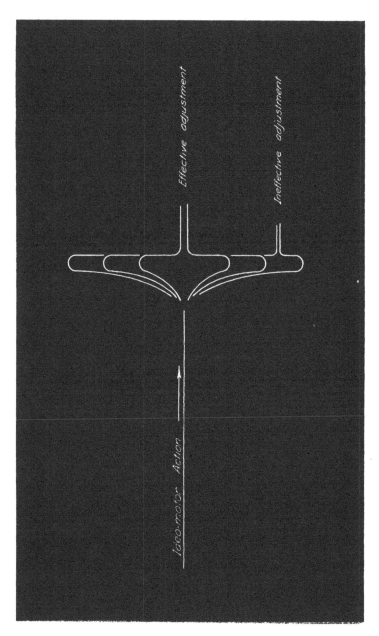

Fig. 12.

[*To face p. 144.*

done either by mental or overt trial and error. Suppose that the craving which demands satisfaction attempts expression in many ways which are all unsuccessful. It is not unreasonable to suppose that the pressure, the demand for and insistence on satisfaction, is thereby increased. If you start a body of water flowing in a certain direction it is a serious matter to stop its flow suddenly. Something may burst if the volume of water and its velocity are sufficient to constitute a considerable momentum. So it is with the mainsprings of our living. In the diagram I have represented this increase of pressure of the motive in successive trials by increasing the width of the section at the point where the consequences of the proposed trial act can be foreseen. As we increase the width of this sector by the increased pressure of the motive there will be more opportunity for the motive to break through in adjustments which would not have constituted the path of least resistance at the initial stages of the drive. It is not unreasonable to suppose that on some occasions the motive will express itself through an adjustment which affords relief in the very immediate perceptual situation, but which does not in the long run satisfy the motive. Such an adjustment would be ineffective when considered in the light of its consequences, but it would be effective in the most immediate sense and it might serve the purpose of draining the motive.

It is a matter of general observation that we are less competent to make keen intelligent judgments when we are wrought up emotionally than when we are in a calm state of mind. Interpreted with reference to the reflex circuit, this would simply mean that when the urgency for an adjustment is not specially severe we can inhibit the expression of the motive at an unfinished ideational stage in order to live through imaginally the remote consequences of the proposed particularization. But this is not so easy when the urgency is severe. This is typically the case when we are emotionally excited. The pressure demanding relief, the urgency for an adaptive adjustment, is then high, and the ideo-motor tendency will then be correspondingly strong. This tendency will particularize and express the motive without the imaginal verification of which we should be capable when the motive is less immediately vital.

Another consideration is the number of available adjustments which increases as the pressure of the motive increases. We do find this in the fact that when we are emotionally excited, when the urgency for an immediate adjustment is strong, we express our motives with many acts in addition to that one act which alone would have constituted the successful adjustment. The pressure spills over, as it were, into adjacent and other actions besides the one which may have been intended. This is typical not only of the situations in which our motivation is excessive but also in those cases in which random trial and error has not yet by habit been reduced to the most effective single and final common path.

Let us consider an illustration. Grant that we all possess gregariousness as one of the main sources of motivation for our conduct. In its ultimate biological sense this motivation may be defended as instinctive, a desire to be accepted by the herd, to have the protection which is afforded by membership in the herd, to be accepted by the strongest and most powerful and influential herd. This instinct is in the case of the human mind a universal demand for the social recognition of our group, of our friends and co-workers, of the general public as far as our social world allows it to be included in our self-concept. Praise, promotion, deference to us, acknowledgment of our necessity and importance, acceptance of us as socially worth-while individuals, satisfy this motive. The failure to get any of these satisfactions makes us restless, unhappy in the place where we are living, critical of everything without knowing the cause, perhaps, arrogant and intolerant in our demands for recognition in the narrow and immediate sense.

During the hours of his job a labourer is perhaps ordered about as though he were a nonentity without self-respect. His work is not made a part of himself. He finds in the shop no opportunity to express and satisfy his own importance, no opportunity to show how clever and capable he thinks he is. This motivation is universal. It applies to every human being. All of us demand first the recognition of those immediately about us. If we fail to get it here in our working environment we transfer our interests and our self-concept to other places where our feeling of worth-whileness is recognized.

If others do not voluntarily recognize and admit our importance we tend to demand it in other direct and indirect ways. We seek then such partial satisfaction as may be obtained in momentary notoriety by our profanity, our unnecessarily bold and aggressive manner, bragging about our achievements which others apparently have not recognized, magnifying trivial situations in which our superiors were at fault or in which they knew less about the job than we did, the situations in which we more or less spectacularly showed how stupid the other fellow was in contrast with us.

Our cravings for recognition break through in more or less ineffective adjustments on those occasions in which we should really rather have our importance voluntarily acknowledged by others. The unsatisfied craving for social approval remains with us and modifies many other adjustments which have at first sight nothing to do with social approval. This is what happens when a man receives a reprimand or some set-back in his work. He inhibits the defensive reply that he would like to give in order not to jeopardize the security of his job, but the dissatisfaction breaks out perhaps in arrogance or arbitrariness against his associates or against the members of his family. This arrogance gives a more or less immediate kind of satisfaction to his craving for social recognition. The recognition is only immediate and it may result in lower esteem afterwards, but it serves nevertheless to relieve the unsatisfied desire in a narrow, temporary, and perceptually immediate sense.

The particular occasion in which we display arrogance in business or at home may involve issues which are quite different from those in which our desire for social approval was frustrated and which brought about our temporary sensitiveness to any sign of lack of approval. Again, this serves to call attention to the futility of trying to describe our mental life in terms of the stimuli or detailed situations in which we act and the particular muscular adjustments which we make. A far more fundamental consideration for the understanding of human nature is to decipher as well as we may the motives that make us act as we do. To describe the stimulus and the response is interesting, but in most cases this is a secondary matter. Such procedure is fruitful only for relatively simple and more or less reflex adjustments.

The satisfaction of our motives is a relative matter. The degree of satisfaction obtained from any given stimulus depends partly on the strength of the motive at the time, and partly on the degree of satisfaction to which we have been accustomed. An unexpected profit of one hundred dollars would affect us differently in relation to our present need for the money on the one hand, and on the other to the amounts of money which we are in the habit of calling our own. It is so with the gregarious instinct. A person who is not accustomed to receive much social approval will be quite elated by a slight encouragement from some source which he considers socially more recognized and more secure than his own. Another man who is accustomed to social approval in more intense form will take the same encouragement as a matter of course.

Another aspect of ineffective adjustment is the over-satiety attained in the satisfaction of a motive that has long remained unsatisfied. A simple case in point is the over-eating which follows starvation for some length of time. The results may actually be detrimental to the fundamental motive which thus expresses itself. Another case of this sort is the so-called " swelled head " of the person who is suddenly advanced to a status which he may long have considered as unattainable. He lives that status with as many as possible of the immediate sorts of satisfaction. He domineers over those who are now under his direction in order to gain the immediate satisfaction which he has tacitly recognized as more or less unattainable. He is not content to take the indirect satisfaction which would be given him for his efficiency in his new position. He wants tangible evidence of his importance here and now. Consequently people must bestir themselves in accordance with his commands at the moment. The same effect can be seen in those who have recently acquired wealth. They must have the visible evidence of their status. It must be perceptually and immediately apparent to themselves and to their friends that thay have attained a financial status with which they have not formerly identified themselves. The man who has been wealthy all his life takes his status for granted. He does not need to show it by his dress, by demanding deference from people about him, by the financial implications of the situations in which people find him. He does not bully the waiter, and he does not mind carrying a package. He is not impelled to demand from the immediate situation the most obvious kind of recognition for his status. He is not slave-bound by the minor social conventions which the newcomer must observe in order to establish his new identity. These cases illustrate how a motive which has not been satisfied for some time acquires more ideo-motor pressure demanding immediate satisfaction than the motive which is more or less habitually released and satisfied.

The same type of behaviour is not infrequently seen with the person who has some kind of inferiority and who over-compensates for it. The inferiority is hardly ever realized consciously. I had occasion recently to see this in two personalities in a garage. One man was the senior partner and the other man was a junior partner. The junior partner was a foreigner who spoke English with a marked accent. The senior partner was an American. I gained the impression repeatedly that the junior partner was the more competent as a mechanic. I had occasion to see them both at work, sometimes on the same problem. The junior partner was nearly always right where there was a difference of opinion. The senior partner would no doubt have been furious if anyone had intimated that he was not so competent a mechanic as his assistant, the foreigner. I am sure that the senior partner did not have the slightest doubt about his superiority, even in his most candid and frank moments of whatever introspection he may have been capable. The two personalities were strikingly different. The junior partner was always courteous, willing to do things for customers, eager to make small repairs in a hurry, if necessary. He never criticized any of his partners in the garage. Occasionally he would give a good-natured smile when his diagnosis proved to be right. The senior partner was a typical grouch. He swore on the slightest provocation, he never had time to do an emergency job, probably on account of a fear of his inability to complete it properly. He criticized the junior partner when the latter was not present. He claimed that his assistant was a drunkard, although I never saw him drunk. The behaviour of the senior partner was in the nature of ineffective expressions of his desire to excel in ability as would behove his status as senior. Failing to get the normal satisfaction of having us recognize his importance, he gained it in a momentary sense by telling us of his own

importance.   He would swear and brag, criticize the
customers for the stupid way in which they handled their cars,
find fault with his assistant on the slightest provocation.
The assistant did not need to be grouchy, because he had
the obvious and tangible satisfaction which came from his
ability to do his work well.   His personality was in consequence well-balanced and good-natured.

There are at least two main factors which determine the
manner in which we express our motives.   These two factors
are the strength of the motive on any occasion and the
habitual manner in which that motive has previously been
expressed.   If the motive is strong it may disrupt the smooth
running of our mental life.   If there is no habitual way in
which the motive may express itself, we may on that account
have some mental disturbance.   We may think of the
breaking of a dam by way of analogy.   There are two main
factors which determinate where the water will run.   The
topography of the land determines the lines of least resistance.
The amount and pressure of the water also determines where
it will go.   If a considerable body of water is suddenly
released from the dam it will not confine itself to the single
channel by which the dam is ordinarily discharged.   The
water will spill over other routes, which are not so low in
level as the principal channel and which were not originally
intended to discharge the water.   So it is with our motives.
If the ideo-motor tendency is strong the motive will discharge not only in the one route which has the lowest
resistance but also in many other routes which have only
relatively low resistance.   If no channel exists at all the
several routes will not differ markedly in their resistance or

level and the discharge will be correspondingly diffuse. This will serve to illustrate that motivation and habit are perhaps primarily responsible for diffuse and unlocalized adjustments. If the motivation is strong there is an increased probability that the adjustments will be diffuse and beyond intelligent control. This is typically the lack of intelligent foresight in extreme emotion. If there are no habits established for the motive the adjustment will tend to be diffuse in the form of random trial and error. This is what we see when a child is learning to write. The motivation has no habitual mode of expression and it issues more or less at random through the facial muscles, the tongue, the feet, and the tightened wrist. With practice these diffuse expressions of the motive disappear and the motivation issues more effectively and completely along those particular lines which by trial and error have been established as effective. A tight wrist in writing or at the piano is therefore properly interpreted as diagnostic of incomplete co-ordination. It shows that the process of defining the motive and limiting it to the most effective final common path has not been completed and that some of the diffused effort of learning is still in evidence. When mastery has been attained the delimitation of the act is completed in the ideational cue instead of overtly.

In order to understand human conduct with any degree of psychological insight, it is necessary to realize the wide range of behaviour in which a basic impulse may express itself. The behaviour is not necessarily rational in any ultimate sense. *One of the basic principles in the interpretation of conduct is that when the impulse is strong, or when it has been frustrated for a considerable time, there is a spread in the type of behaviour by which the impulse expresses itself.* Since the impulse is denied satisfaction in the behaviour which is natural and normal, it seeks satisfaction in substitute conduct which by superficial appearance may be entirely irrelevant and inappropriate. The effect corresponds to the random behaviour by which an impulse expresses itself in the early stages of learning.

Another basic principle in the interpretation of conduct is that when the satisfactions for which an impulse is striving are denied, there is a restriction in temporal reference to the immediate present. By this is meant that an impulse may seek satisfaction in behaviour which is adequate when viewed from the standpoint of the immediate moment, even though it may be entirely inadequate and obviously ineffective when viewed from the standpoint of its permanent or future effects. A very common example is the provocation for swearing and bragging as expressions of self-advancement and the desire for superiority. The satisfaction may be attained momentarily, although it is not permanently effective. This principle is in line with the principle that we have previously discussed regarding the temporal reference of intelligent and unintelligent conduct. *The more intelligent the conduct, the more remote is the expected benefit.*

In our discussion of autistic and realistic thinking we found occasion to say that the autistic form of thought is not always and necessarily harmful. Only its extreme indulgence is to be discouraged. We should make the same conclusion regarding certain varieties of ineffective adjustment. Ineffective adjustments should not necessarily and always be discouraged merely because they are ineffective in the normal and more or less enduring sense. *If an impulse is strong and if it has been denied its normal satisfaction, there are occasionally situations in which the peace of mind and the balance of the personality can be more readily retained by giving vent to the unsatisfied impulse through ineffective behaviour that gives only momentary release, even though the momentary ineffective behaviour is entirely irrational and useless from the standpoint of outside observers.* Such is the case with a sudden burst of profanity, or with a crying spell, when they are expressions of a suddenly blocked impulse or desired state. To inhibit the momentary release of the impulse can be the cause of a strain on the personality for hours or days. Explosive behaviour is not intelligent, and it is not social, but it has a value for the individual which must not be overlooked. Since the development of personality is essentially in the direction of social acceptability, it should be clear that the extensive reliance on the momentary release of our impulses is socially detrimental as well as permanently ineffective, but, on the other hand, we should not make the mistake of branding all explosive and ineffective behaviour as useless.

CHAPTER XII

A DEFINITION OF INTELLIGENCE

1. *Intelligence as incompleteness of expected behaviour*
2. *Consummatory behaviour*
3. *Animal intelligence*
4. *A child's intelligence*
5. *Adult intelligence*

1. INTELLIGENCE AS INCOMPLETENESS OF EXPECTED BEHAVIOUR

We started our discussion of intelligent and non-intelligent behaviour with the assumption that conduct originates in the organism itself and that it is only secondarily determined by the environment. With this assumption we place the stimulus in the rôle of a modifier of intended conduct, or as the medium through which self-expression takes place. We look for causal factors beyond the stimulus—in the organism itself—and it is in the impulses of the inner self that we must find the datum for psychology. We find that this point of view is implied or stated by most of the writers in the field of abnormal psychology, and that it is not the point of view represented by most of the scientific psychologists. We have described various aspects of this fundamental process of self-expression, one aspect of which constitutes what we know as intelligence. It is now our purpose to summarize these observations about the reflex circuit into a definition of intelligence which shall be consistent with the point of view that we have outlined. Such definitions we have already given as parts of the discussion of related topics, but we shall summarize them here with special regard to what we know as different degrees or levels of intelligence.

We assume, first of all, that there is a continuum between the impulses that constitute the inner self, the conscious life that is present to introspection, and the behaviour for which consciousness is the natural preparation. These three phases of the psychological act terminate in what we know as the overt act or overt behaviour. We postulate a functional identity of the three phases of the psychological act, in that consciousness is assumed to be made of the same stuff that behaviour is made of. Consciousness is incomplete behaviour. Mental states constitute conduct which is in the process of being formed. The sequence from the impulses that constitute the inner self to the behaviour by which satisfactions are to be attained is primarily one of delimitation. In the early phase of the circuit, the impulse is relatively vague, unlocalized, diffuse, universal. At the terminal or overt phase it is relatively definite, localized, specific, and particular.

The psychological differentiæ for the several levels of the psychological act relate to the degree of definition of the impulse. Those states of mind in which the impulse is as yet only loosely specified are known as universals. They are the higher thought processes. Those states of mind in which the expected experience is relatively well specified

are known as perception or as the simpler ideational processes. The higher thought processes differ from the simpler
ideational processes mainly in the degree of definition of the
expected adjustment.

It should be evident that if the act is made focal when it
is as yet only a universal, there is ample opportunity to
specify the details over a wide range of behaviour. If, on
the other hand, the act is made focal when it is almost
completely specified, there is considerable restriction in the
range of behaviour through which it may be finally expressed.
This greater latitude of choice over a wide range of possible
types of adjustment constitutes the biological advantage
of the higher thought processes. We have discussed this
characteristic of the reflex circuit also with regard to overt
and mental trial and error. The higher thought processes
have been described as a trial-and-error process that is
carried out with loosely organized and tentative alternatives,
whereas the perceptual and overt forms of trial and error
are carried out with alternatives that are already closely
specified. They leave little latitude for further choice.

The focal point in the reflex circuit we have defined as
that stage in the expression of an impulse at which the
impulse becomes conscious. The impulse may become focal
when it is almost ready to precipitate into overt action, or
it may become focal while it is still only a vague, loosely
organized desire. In the latter case the impulse contains
relatively few attributes when it becomes focal, whereas in
the former case it is already specified as to most of its details.
That part of the reflex circuit which temporally precedes
the focus of consciousness is called the preconscious.

The part of the reflex circuit which succeeds the focus of consciousness is subject to introspective description. It is characteristic of the preconscious phase of the circuit that it is not subject to observation and inhibitive control.

The intelligence of any particular psychological act is a function of the incomplete stage of the act at which it is the subject of trial-and-error choice. Intelligence, considered as a mental trait, is the capacity to make impulses focal at their early, unfinished stage of formation. Intelligence is therefore the capacity for abstraction, which is an inhibitory process. In the intelligent moment the impulse is inhibited while it is still only partially specified, while it is still only loosely organized. It is then known as a universal or a concept. The trial-and-error choice and elimination, in intelligent conduct, is carried out with alternatives that are so incomplete and so loosely organized that they point only toward types of behaviour without specifying the behaviour in detail.

2. CONSUMMATORY BEHAVIOUR

In the lowest form of conduct that we can imagine with regard to its intelligence, we have every impulse of the organism expressed in purely random forms without consciousness. It is purely reflex. In such behaviour every impulse expresses itself without inhibition or anticipation of the experience. Such random behaviour is continued until the satisfactions of the organism are attained. The life of such organisms is limited entirely to contact experience of the consummatory sort. Consciousness implies anticipation of experience and that is impossible in a life that is limited to consummatory and random contact experience.

3. ANIMAL INTELLIGENCE

The first sign of intelligence appears when the consummatory contact experience is associated with sense-experience. After a few repetitions of such association the sense-experience alone comes to represent the completion of the experience. The sense-impression comes to mean the expected consummation in contact form. The trial-and-error elimination of failures is then removed from the realm of completely enacted contact experience to the realm in which these contact experiences are merely indicated by their corresponding sensory cues. The impulses that are checked in terms of the expected experience, with which the sensory cues of the moment have been associated, are said to be conscious. Consciousness is, functionally considered, just this expectation of a completed experience in terms of the indices of the moment. It implies a shift of the trial-and-error life of the actor from overt experience to the incomplete experience which is the sensory cue. This has been shown to be essentially a process of conditioning in the behaviouristic sense. Animal intelligence is limited in the degree of incompleteness of expected experience at which its trial-and-error life may be carried out. It is limited in its capacity for abstraction to that degree of it which is marked by the use of sensory cues as indices of expected experience. Its trial-and-error choice of behaviour is therefore limited to the immediate present.

4. A CHILD'S INTELLIGENCE

If we continue the progress marked by the shift of the trial-and-error point from among overt particulars to the stage at which these particulars are anticipated in terms of the sensory cues, we come to the stage of development of mind at which the actor can make focal his impulses for trial-and-error choice in the absence of the stimulus. That is ideation. It is directly continuous with the intelligence that is limited to the immediate present. This further progress simply means that the impulse is made focal at a still less defined stage when it has still fewer attributes, being stripped even of those attributes which are implied by the sensory cue.

The intelligence of the child is greatly in advance of that of the animal in that it is able to anticipate experience which is not perceptually present. The child is capable of ideational trial and error even though the process is for a time limited to the situations in which perceptual experience is imaginally represented rather than universals of higher order. The child's imagination is limited to the situations in which its bodily relations are imaginally specified. It remains for the intelligence level of the adult to be able to imagine expected experience so incompletely specified that one's bodily relations are not imaginally represented.

5. ADULT INTELLIGENCE

In the normal adult intelligence we have the capacity to represent expected experience in terms of cues that point toward types of experience and in which the bodily relations of the actor are not even specified. This is conceptual thinking. The types of experience are represented in conceptual thinking by symbols that are less detailed than the perceptual cues. The visual and auditory images that serve as indices of meaning in the adult mind are in reality incomplete acts which are being accepted or rejected in terms of the purposes of the moment. The meaning of a concept is the potential particularization of the imaginal cue into expected experience.

We have seen that the differentiation of the exploring function of the receptors is the beginning of the development of intelligence. The biological function of intelligence is to protect the organism from bodily risk and to satisfy its wants with the least possible chance of recording failure on the environment. This is accomplished by deflecting an impulse which is headed toward failure before the failure is realized. It is made possible by the fact that, psychologically, a part of an experience serves the purpose of guiding the whole of the experience. The percept represents the experience that would be met if the percept were ignored. The deflection of an impulse toward or away from an experience is determined by that small part of the experience which constitutes the sensory cue or its ideational equivalent. If a certain course of action is declared to be a bad policy and thereby rejected, the future failure is eliminated when the impulse is only conceptual and before the details of the impending failure have been realized.

In a biological sense the higher thought processes serve the same purpose for the organism as the simplest anatomical differentiation of the exploring function. The two are exactly the same in kind. They differ only in the degree of incompleteness of the experiences that are being chosen and eliminated.

It is of some interest to speculate about the nature of the continued development of intelligence. Further development of intelligence might give facility in selecting effective behaviour with impulses that are close to their source, while they are in what we know as the preconscious or subconscious. To think would then be to use terms that are less and less cognitive but more and more loaded with affectivity. It might possibly come about that the highest possible form of intelligence is one in which the alternatives are essentially nothing but affective states. Some characteristics of genius would not be inconsistent with such a view.

SUMMARY

In closing, it should be pointed out that the interpretation of mind, and particularly of intelligence, that these chapters represent is not in all particulars novel, because it is at least implied in current psychological discussion. The contribution is primarily in calling attention to the possible fruitfulness, for the understanding of human conduct, of an attitude of inquiry concerning the satisfactions that normal people seek. It is in this direction that we shall probably find the most illuminating facts concerning human nature and conduct. That the environment is an extremely essential factor in determining conduct is, of course, obvious. The point that I am stressing in many different ways is that when we are studying human nature, either in the laboratory or in our daily lives, it is much more conducive to psychological insight to look for the satisfactions that people seek through their conduct, than to judge them as merely responding to a more or less fortuitous environment. The case cannot rest solely on the degree of accuracy of description because either point of view lends itself fairly well to accurate description of conduct. The case will be decided by the relative success of the two attitudes. It is my belief that the attitude, which is implied in the so-called new psychology, has given, in a relatively short space of time, more insight into human conduct than the thoroughly objective point of view which has in recent years become established in scientific psychology, and which has been borrowed from related objective sciences.

Our interpretation of consciousness as incomplete behaviour, and our placement of the sources of conduct in the inner self, should have ramifications in the fields of ethics, education, and esthetics. Morals should be a legitimate subject-matter for psychology, not in the superficial sense of merely establishing " bonds " between available stimuli and the behaviour that is declared to be expedient, but in a much more human way in which social conduct and non-social conduct are understood as expressing conflicts of a self. This is the modern tendency in the interpretation of crime and other deviations from the conventional codes. Why should not psychological studies be furthered with a point of view that has been found effective in actually dealing with human conduct ? Is it not a handicap to change our point of view when we pass from the situations in which we actually deal with conduct to the situations in which we attempt to formulate it with academic and scientific precision ?

In the field of education our interpretation should prove particularly applicable. A brand of educational psychology is being taught to prospective teachers in which they are drilled in the jargon of establishing " bonds " between stimuli and the desired behaviour. It would be more appropriate to describe the normal impulses of children, and the methods by which children may be induced to express these impulses in ways that are profitable. Again, the accuracy of description is not the criterion by which a choice of interpretation should be made, because both of them work for descriptive purposes. Take, as an example, the troublesome question of interest in students. If we assume that the child naturally seeks satisfactions that are typical for its age and maturity, we shall find interest to be merely the relevancy of the environment to the wants that originate in the child. A stimulus that does not serve as a tool for the child's satisfaction, as seen by the child, is simply not a stimulus. It is not attended to. The central problem of interest is, therefore, first of all, to list the desires of children and the numerous ways in which these desires may be satisfied. It is the teacher's task to use the innate desire of the child as the motive power for its own work, and to make available those stimuli which the child normally seeks and which also serve the instructional purposes. If a lesson is not so arranged that it serves as an avenue of natural self-expression for the child, there is no internal motive power to make the child think, and the teacher is thereby increasing her own labours. These facts may be accurately described with the stimulus-response jargon, but the teacher who is so equipped does not develop insight into the causal factors at work in the child's mind. That teacher is more fortunate who realizes that the starting-point for the educative process is in the child's own mind, and that the tools of education are merely the means whereby we attempt to induce the child to express its own self in a direction that may be ultimately advantageous.

I hope, further, that the consistent interpretation of mental phenomena as conduct in the process of being formed, and the interpretation of every mental state as incomplete action, will assist to some extent in unifying the several schools of psychology which are now talking totally different languages. The structuralist and the functionalist devote themselves to mental states as such, the behaviourist confines himself to behaviour that can be physically seen and measured, the psychiatrist is primarily interested in the subconscious sources of queer conduct. The content of these three main types of psychological inquiry constitutes, according to our present interpretation, the three phases of a continuum. Conduct would be thought of as starting in the obscure sources of the inner self which psychiatrists are studying. These sources become impulses as introspectively known to the conscious self. They are now studied by the academic schools of psychology as though they were more or less distinct entities. These impulses, as consciously known, would be thought of as conflicts which are being decided while the contestants are still unexpressed in conduct. The behaviour, and the cessation of behaviour that accompanies satisfaction, would be thought of, not as the exclusive and only possible subject-matter for psychology, but rather as the biological objective for which mind does its work. In a certain sense, our interpretation is behaviouristic, because behaviour is the centre about which the mental antecedents are interpreted, and yet behaviour is, after all, only a means to an end in the satisfactions that we seek. *Psychology starts with the unrest of the inner self, and it completes its discovery in the contentment of the inner self.* Only with such an interpretation can human psychology be considered to be human. With it, also, we are able to follow with genuine interest the medical, psychological, and behaviouristic studies that throw light on the causal factors in human conduct.